D0065922

UN
BOTHERED

OMARION

UN
BOTHERED

THE POWER OF CHOOSING JOY

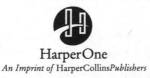

HarperOne

An Imprint of HarperCollins*Publishers*

HarperCollins books may be purchased for educational, business, or sales promotional use. For information, please email the Special Markets Department at SPsales@harpercollins.com.

FIRST EDITION

Designed by Elina Cohen

Illustration © Oprah Woode

Library of Congress Cataloging-in-Publication Data is available upon request.

ISBN 978-0-06-311918-5

22 23 24 25 26 LSC 10 9 8 7 6 5 4 3 2 1

CONTENTS

PART 3 MENTAL

FOREWORD

Omarion is a great spirit full of creativity and enthusiasm. You might know him mostly as a singer, dancer, and actor; however, beyond those roles, Omarion is a Truth seeker and a Truth teller. I had the joy of working with Omarion on a project to raise funds for the nonprofit MusiCares during the COVID-19 pandemic at one of Agape's online services. It included offering a musical challenge to folks to sing Bill Withers's seminal song, "Lovely Day," as a way to help lift people's spirits. I discovered at the time that Omarion had been following my teachings and had a spiritual practice of his own. During our interview and dialogue, it was clear to me that Omarion was more than an entertainer: he was and is a disciple of Spiritual truth who seeks to live his life in accordance with Spiritual principles. Like most of us, Omarion's life experiences have been both very wonderful and very challenging. However, it is his deep Spiritual longing that has allowed him to unfold into his own unique expression of inspiration and upliftment, as demonstrated by his latest creative offering, *Unbothered: The Power of Choosing Joy*. To be "unbothered" is to live in a high state of mind and consciousness. It does not mean being indifferent to, ignoring, tuning out, or avoiding our thoughts, emotions, and feelings, especially during challenging times, which we as men have a tendency to do, but having the mental, emotional, and spiritual tools and resources to better understand them and navigate through our life experiences and relationships in self-loving and self-affirming ways, regardless of any circumstance. In fact and in Truth, no matter what problems, challenges, or even crises we experience that might grab hold of our hearts and minds, our Souls, the Spiritual core essence of who and what we are, remain untouched (and unbothered) because Spirit only knows the high vibration of Love, peace, compassion, clarity, joy, generosity, freedom, grace, abundance, and beauty. What's more, It constantly beckons us, calling us home to align with that Truth of our being, which we can access at any time we choose to. See, Life loves us so much that It built within each of us an unwavering support and guidance system that is always available to us. Through his Spiritual practice, Omarion has learned how to tap into that in ways that have allowed him to move through and transcend personal challenges and emerge with the wisdom learned and earned through insight and inspiration. And in *Unbothered* his readers benefit from the lessons and takeaways of his journey, which offer tools and principles on how to do the same, as well as navigate the inevitable ups and downs of life with more ease and grace. If you have ever had questions about how to live your life with more purpose, happiness, and resiliency, this book is your answer. In-joy the journey it takes you on.

Peace and Richest Blessings,

Michael B. Beckwith
Founder and CEO, Agape International
Spiritual Center
Author, *Life Visioning* and *Spiritual Liberation*

A NOTE ON YANTRAS: THE SACRED SYMBOL ANCHORING THIS BOOK

At the beginning of each meditation, you will find yantras: sacred symbols used as visual tools for meditation in Hinduism and Buddhism. A yantra is composed of geometric shapes generating a subtle range of cosmic forces matching the invoked energy. The O yantra that appears throughout this book works with divine vibrations to connect to the energies of the divine, illuminating positive energies and destroying negative energies, which can help an individual elevate spiritually. This particular yantra has an enso circle within it—this is a sacred symbol in Zen Buddhism representing the circle of togetherness. The enso has a special meaning to me because of its spiritual roots and its mirror to my name. I hope that it helps you in your practice as it has for me.

INTRODUCTION

I take pride in being who I say I am, in and out of the public eye. Being unbothered is more than just a catchy saying or a fitting title. It's truly my way of life. When I think about my growth as a man, and my ability to persevere, greet adversity head-on, and be unswayed by negativity, everything feels like it's come full circle. I didn't get to where I am overnight. I've practiced and worked hard to reach this level of maturity. Over the years, my life has come full circle. Enso is a sacred symbol in Zen Buddhism meaning *circle* or, sometimes, *circle of togetherness*. I feel aligned with the power that the enso shape holds. Like me, it is more than what meets the eye. Being unbothered is a sacred practice. It serves as a reminder that I am surrounded by wholeness and protection no matter what comes my way. My ability to live an unbothered life is connected to a deeper meaning. To be unbothered, to me, means to be grounded and connected to your truth. No one can shake or destroy a foundation that is built on solid ground. I look at being unbothered as a lifestyle and daily practice of protecting my peace and energy. We have a choice in how we react and respond. I have been evolving into my entire and highest self since the beginning of my career. A lot has unfolded for me over the years. A lot of things have come together too. I've grown as a man, become a father to two beautiful children, and I've done my best to figure out how to be a man of integrity, good character, and honesty. *Unbothered* represents my growth as a man, father, musician, and human being—getting it right and getting it wrong. You'll find some of my greatest lessons and takeaways in this book. From how I uncovered my purpose to my thoughts on being happy and whole, even when adversity strikes, you'll get to know me and my story on a new level and in a new way. I'll be sharing intimate thoughts with you about things I've grown to understand on a deeper level, like energy exchange, fear, love, and legacy. There are tools throughout the book that have helped me at my lowest point and supported me at my highest. Meditations, mantras, and affirmations have been game changers as I move through the world in ways that are intentional. We all seek wholeness in our lives and our experiences. I've come to realize that over time, wholeness can look and feel different, and that is okay.

Over the years, I've been deeply inspired by teachers like Dr. Michael Beckwith. His work and mission have shown me how to grow closer to myself mentally and spiritually. I was first introduced to Dr. Beckwith through my brother O'Ryan. After some major life changes, I started practicing yoga and learning how to control my thoughts and emotions. Dr. Beckwith welcomed me with open arms into Agape, his Spiritual Center for community building, love, and embodiment of evolving consciousness. In my experience with Dr. Beckwith and his teachings, I understand the importance of how I act and speak as it pertains to the way I respond to life and its challenges. I share this because I've found great peace in staying connected and committed to having ease in my life—and I find joy and purpose in sharing my life lessons and takeaways with you all. People joke about me being the Unbothered King; but all jokes aside, it's taken me years of self-reflection and evolution to get to where I am today. No one is an overnight success. Everyone has their own unique journey and path to embark on. Transformation hasn't been easy. Changing and growing while being in the public eye is even more challenging. However, as I look back on my life and into my future, my growth as a man has been a full-circle experience. In the pages of this book, you'll see that through my highs and my lows. My hope is that you resonate with them and take away your own lessons and practices. The wisdom that comes with life, heartbreak, business, and change is where we learn to piece together the things in our lives that leave us feeling broken, stuck, or unsure. This book is an invitation to lean in and learn how you want to create the life you want.

Unbothered is more than a book. If you're looking for a B2K tell-all, or to get a glimpse into the details of my romantic relationships, this isn't for you. *Unbothered* is a tool for those ready to learn what it means to stand in their power through hardship and joy. It's for those looking at what it truly means to live unbothered and unswayed by distractions. I know that life isn't always easy or fair. It can come at us fast and, at times, will knock us on our ass. But we were built for this soul work: we're made to change and become better. On this journey, people will let us down and try to distract us from our calling, but when we are focused on our destiny and aware of our truth, nothing can get in the way of the greatness we're destined to achieve. No one can take away from the legacies we're making. My hope is that this collection of lessons and takeaways will serve as a reminder that no matter what comes our way, we have the power of choice. We have the ability to rise in integrity and dignity despite the challenges or pain we face. I've chosen to live my life with self-understanding at the heart of everything I do. While I am not without flaws, I am committed to doing and being my best. I am focused on what matters most, and that's staying true to my purpose and character.

The definition of full circle is *a series of developments that lead back to the original source.* We are the original source. There is power in that! Everything that comes our way can and will teach us something if we're open to observing, listening, and becoming better. True life is lived. And as a Spanish proverb explains, "A wise man changes his mind, a fool never will." Dare to shine bright in a world full of darkness. Being deeply rooted in your purpose will create new air around you. It'll remind you to explore the whys in your life and encourage you to stay on a path of enlightenment when it comes to the things you're setting out to achieve. I read a quote that has stuck with me: "You have power over your mind—not outside events—that is where you find strength." Let this body of work serve as a reminder of collective resilience and responsibility for ourselves and others. Be *unbothered*; you were made for this. Don't doubt your ability to bring your life full circle—you are worthy of everything good that you call in, so make room.

—*O.*

PART 1 |

SPIRITUAL

1

Purpose

It's in my nature, as a man, to show up in the spaces I occupy, and in my family, as a protector—as a person who is present, intentional, and mindful of the moves I make and the words I speak. Everything has meaning and place. Everything is a pillar or a key to something. It's essential for me to remember and acknowledge my truth as I grow and change. My purpose is ever-changing and unfolding, and a lot of people don't talk about that. There are many layers to who we are as people, and I find that to be true about the purpose, or the many purposes, we have in life. Standing steadfast in what I am here for and what I've been called to do serves as the foundation of my existence. It also offers clarity when I've been challenged and in moments of reflection. *What am I here for?* is a question that I ask myself when greeted with change or a moment of choice. I'm a creator, dancer, father, protector, and so much more.

Each outlet is connected to my purpose. Being multifaceted is beautiful, and I feel the most grounded in a purpose-driven life when I tap into the different parts and passions of mine. Every decision that we make in life is linked to an outcome, good or bad, supportive of our journeys or hurtful. Knowing our purpose, or having a curiosity about what it could be, allows us to be flexible and continue to be students of life. So even when we make mistakes and don't get it right, there's room for us to lean in, get curious, and create an inner dialogue as we consider our behavior, talents, and lives as a whole. Knowing who we are, or at least getting curious about who we can be, plays a major role in who we end up being in this life.

YOU'RE HERE FOR A REASON. SHARE YOUR GIFTS.

Being clear about my purpose has shifted many things, like how I move through relationships, romance, fatherhood, and my career. After many years of reflection and growth, I've also come to realize that my purpose chose me. Long before I could imagine my calling, it was already written in the stars. It existed inside me, patiently waiting for me to take notice and say *yes* to it. I got signs along the way that would present themselves. A powerful lesson for me on my pathway to purpose has been understanding that at some point, to truly live fully, we have to be brave, fearless, and self-aware enough to recognize what is calling for our attention and care. We are required to take action as we explore what comes to the surface by being open to the possibility of being greater than we already are. What we answer to and how we show up in this life for those around us is directly linked to our life's work and what we're called to do. The work that we do for others is a direct reflection of the work we desire for ourselves. We are each other's mirror. When I realized that my existence on earth wasn't by accident, I could clearly see the benefit in how my actions and behavior affected those around me. My purpose has been the cornerstone to support the legacy that will remain long after I'm gone. Even in the face of adversity, conflict, or fear, being mindful about intentions, answering the calling of my heart's work, is proof that we'll get what we put out.

EVERYTHING WILL
COME FULL CIRCLE IN
THE END. STAY PATIENT
AND CONNECTED TO
YOUR TRUTH.

The art of creating is being able to accept the things that come toward you versus running away from them. Receiving what comes your way with open arms can speak to your energetic vibration. I am very in tune with energy, which means I can identify when things feel aligned and meant for me. When you are open to receiving, your vibration is high, you feel safe, you feel grounded, and you learn to pay attention to what is speaking for and through you. A high-energetic vibration makes room for tapping into the lesson and information that you need to see your higher self. I've chosen to pay attention to the signs presented to me. Two signs continue to come up in my life: that my music affects people—it is central to some of their important memories and it can reflect an emotion they can't express on their own—and that my music creates a connection between myself and others: there is something spectacular about being connected to people I've never met through my music.

One moment stands out clearly in my mind. Many years ago, before the internet and social media, when being on the radio was everything, I was doing an interview. This girl called in, excited to talk with me, and shared a story that I'll never forget. She told me that "Ice Box" was her and her best friend's favorite song. That friend had passed away. She shared that they buried a picture of me with him and that those memories of the love for my music will forever be cherished, remembered, and appreciated. It was humbling to hear her recall this. It stopped me in my tracks and made me realize that music is the truest form of connection and love. From then on, I understood that I was a bridge in their experience by way of music, and many others carry similar experiences. It's moments like that that remind me of what I was put on this earth to do. It's moments like that one that will live in my heart forever and serve as a frequent reminder of the expansiveness of purpose and the power of music. When you recognize your purpose, you can fill your soul. A part of serving your soul is helping others. My work, this work, *is* purpose work. Even if I wanted to, there'd be no way to ignore the significance of showing up and taking the lead. If we allow ourselves to be open, we make space for receiving what is meant to be ours.

| Energy Check: Purpose

What are you willing to struggle for?

What activity makes you forget about the world around you?

If you have a dream, could you bring it into reality?

What's your motivation style?

What gives meaning to your life?

There were moments on this journey where I questioned if I could handle the responsibility of submitting to my purpose. *Could I take it? What would I do in moments where the goodness of life seemed clouded? Could I accept it?* The unknown proved to be frightening, but I wasn't willing to ignore it and not see what was in store for me. There will be mistakes made along the way. Self-discovery requires missteps. That's where the lessons are hidden. As humans, we fuck up. How we honor our process and right our wrongs is a part of the journey. There are so many things we don't have control over. Fear will sometimes present itself as an obstacle, and even still, our life's work and purpose will remain steadfast and waiting for us to move forward, scared or not. We have to overcome to grow. Doing things scared can be the fertile ground for immense growth and self-discovery. Letting fear be the ruler of our lives cannot be an option. We all know from experience that fear can and will hold us back and hostage if we let it. Being and staying committed to living an expansive life, no matter what tries to stop us, is how we build our muscles of resilience and perseverance.

From a young age, I knew what I wanted: I wanted to be an Entertainer and to creatively express myself through my art. I've been committed to my art since before I can remember. This commitment took me to the highest heights of the entertainment industry. But it also tested my connection to my own inner voice, because fame has a curious way of distracting you from what really matters. B2K had been together for four years, and people had known Omarion, JBoog, Raz-B, and Fizz as a unit. When B2K broke up, it may have appeared to the outside world that my purpose was in jeopardy. But instead, parting ways prepared me for a new sense of self-belief, living intentionally and being more open than ever to pave a new path for myself as a solo artist. It was a new beginning and a new chance to connect with my original purpose: being an Entertainer. The first thing I needed to do was to expand my territory and extend my reach creatively, but that meant going from performing in front of tens of thousands of people to small crowds in nightclubs and intimate settings for royal families in faraway places. It was humbling. It felt like I was tired of the performance life. It took a lot out of me physically and emotionally. I was forced out of my comfort zone—and it was through discomfort that I started looking at my destiny as a musician and performer in a new way. I am always looking for more ways to grow and become better. That's the personality that I have. Being average isn't an option, and neither is quitting. I was committed to trusting my process and staying true to my intentions of touching hearts and changing lives with my music and message. These small actions built on themselves, creating new ground for myself. I had to step back in order to move forward. This required a mental reset, refocusing and pivoting toward my next level.

The most powerful moment I had during this period, after many sleepless nights, show after show, was performing for the Aboriginal people in Australia on Indigenous land. Going overseas to perform was always an adventure. And I mean that quite literally. When I stepped out of the car in Alice Springs, Australia, the brutal heat greeted me and nothing was what I was accustomed to. The crowd and the venue were small and unembellished with its 4x8 stage and modest sound system. This was entirely new territory for me because I was in an unfamiliar place with otherwise unacceptable circumstances. I had to humble myself to experience it fully. A part of me wanted to not be there at all, but going home wasn't an option because in order to break new ground, I needed to get uncomfortable. There was a difference between being a star in the US and an international star, and I had to remind myself of that, even if it meant that my first shows abroad weren't stadiums. My goal was to have my music touch as many people as and as many hearts as possible. Yes, I was frustrated after getting out of the car and seeing what I had to work with because nothing was what I was used to back in the States and rightfully so. It wasn't supposed to be the same. This was new territory for me, and regardless of the circumstance, this small group of people was looking for me to show up and perform. So I got myself together and did my job because no matter how big or small the crowd, my goal was to both affect and inspire others, even if it's just one person, and to continue my own path of reinvention as an artist. Keeping this as my center enabled me to transform what it means to be an entertainer during this pivotal time in my life. Driving through the mountains in Australia to perform for people who were unfamiliar with me and vice versa was eye-opening to my true purpose. We didn't speak the same language, but we all could relate through music. It was a trip to see how far and deep the vibration of merely being human connected us. After the performance, I did a meet and greet for the small group of people I had just performed for. It was then that I learned what it truly meant to be bound by music. The ability to share new experiences, stories, and visions is what being alive is all about. We all need that. No matter how outside of my comfort zone I may have felt in the beginning, by the end, the purpose of the trip and the experience as a whole became very clear. Humans were created to connect. The status, success, and societal symbols of greatness do not make us who we are. They do not deepen our connections to those around us.

This wisdom about what matters in life might sound obvious to some—wise men have taught this for millennia—but practicing it is a different story. As someone who grew up onstage and in the media from a young age, I had a lot to unlearn about what makes me a person of value. By the time I went solo, I had a crash course in what my priorities were and how I defined success. Society likes to tell us how successful we are when, really, success is a perspective. I've had number ones. I've gotten plaques. I've been nominated for a Grammy. And in my reflection, all of that has made room for me to ask what does this all mean? In truth, it's in the small moments, the starting from the ground up moments, that we genuinely find camaraderie and deep understanding for those around us. Accolades and acknowledgment are important to an extent, but there comes a time when life has to matter beyond the praise you receive. Life is about more than having influence and power. Your gifts weren't given to you for the sole purpose of being seen and accepted by the masses. No matter what they are, our talents are bridges for human connection to cross and meet in the middle. To create something for the world to be a better place. This speaks to something more extraordinary outside ourselves. It is a testament to divine purpose over profit. That is the real influence. Being taken away from my audience in the States and thrust into foreign territory taught me to expand and mature as a performer and genuinely anchor into being open to new experiences.

It was during this time after B2K ended and I launched my solo career that I also deepened the spiritual path I was on. My Nana taught my brother and I at an early age how to connect with Spirit. The first thing I started doing differently was praying. Then I started practicing gratitude and being present with what was around me and in front of me. My goal was to become freer in my life and more connected with my creativity. All these things play a part in what I was able to achieve during this evolution. By finding centeredness, I found my authentic and creative voice.

In the music business, it means something to have awards, be on lists, and get plaques. And while those things are nice milestone moments, they don't *make* me great. Staying responsible for my success and the imprint I leave on the world is what makes my greatness not only expansive but authentic and aligned with the highest good of my life. Artists can get tricked into thinking that we aren't valuable if the crowds aren't filling arenas, if the records aren't selling, or if our music isn't streaming by the millions if we aren't topping the charts. That is a dangerous mirage that can swallow a person whole and manipulate the true purpose at hand. And when I was thousands of miles away from home, in a tiny Australian town that I never knew existed, the truth, my truth, became even more evident. No matter your life walk, we all have moments of feeling displaced and lost. You can uncover your purpose no matter who you are or where you came from.

The road to success is long. It requires failures and missteps because it is there that we learn what lessons to take with us as we continue to press forward. When you're curious about your purpose, when your intentions are transparent, open, and honest, they will link up. You become a force that no one can stop. My goal has always been to change the world as an artist by inspiring people with my music. That small town in Australia opened up a new pathway to a deeper meaning for me. I walked away with a more explicit connection to what it means to live guided by what I was called to do in this life.

I'm constantly reminded that I'm a thinker, and I'm also someone who enjoys life's everyday things. Reflecting on my time in Australia is a beautiful reminder of the blessings that I'm able to experience every day. Some people forget that I am a human being, not just a celebrity who gets things done for them—I do my own grocery shopping and pump my own gas. But because of how the world sees famous people, it's almost like folks expect me to live up to a certain worldly projection. No one looked at me in that way when I was overseas, and it was refreshing. I was able to show up and do my job without the extra stuff attached. When I think about living my purpose, I grow more and more aware that I'm being met with other people's perspectives and perceptions—through all that I have to stay grounded in who I am and what I've been chosen to do while on this planet.

Being a celebrity meant that I risked losing sight of my own inner voice and motivations early in my career, but my experiences in going solo helped me to stay close to my inner truth. I experienced the gift of tapping into my first passion for artistic projects and into a newfound interest in truth seeking for a long time after this period. My purpose started when I was performing in the living room as a young kid. Creativity was my driving force. Yet my purpose has continued to transform in my life with the various responsibilities of what it means to be a man. Today I live two different lives, a public life that I consider my job and a regular family guy life that offers me the time and space to take care of my business as a man moving through the world with a family and other responsibilities. Living in my purpose has put me in a position to see other people's perspectives and perceptions—whether or not I understand or can relate. I think that purpose has a way of shifting your perspective. In all that I do in my life, I like to be intentional. I feel that I am most effective no matter where I am and what I'm doing.

My mom having me at sixteen really informed who I was

growing up. She was a child having a child, but even with that being true, we got to grow up together in a cool way. My mom poured herself into me as a child, and she played a significant role in molding me into who I am today. She told me I could be whoever and whatever I wanted to be. I think that her being young and ambitious herself played a significant role in that messaging. My relationship with my mom was very different from the relationships I saw my friends having with their parents. I remember my mom being such a go-getter and hard worker, no matter what obstacles presented themselves. She wasn't quitting or giving up. She was a hairstylist when I was growing up. She did everyone's hair, from executives to folks singing in God's Property with Kirk Franklin. I was around for all of it—always in the mix. My brother and I were always on set, at shoots, and witnessing our mother stand in her purpose without fear. When I really look back on my purpose, it was being cultivated at a young age. I was already in a position to shape my gift. I never felt the pressure to become anything because being creative and great was already being led by an example. It didn't matter if I wanted to dance, sing, or play basketball. Whatever I said I wanted to do, my mom facilitated it. That support was the breeding ground for my purpose of being what it is today.

Another critical thing that nurtured my purpose as a protector was growing up around my Nana. She kept us close to our culture and identity. I remember going to an event back in the day called the African Marketplace. It was at the high school my mom went to, Dorsey High. I also filmed my first national commercial there, so there was a great synergy and sense of belonging when we would go. Being around that type of energy helped nurture my creativity. I grew up with the community, immediate, and extended family all around, so I was always supported and encouraged to be myself. It was a blessing to never feel the pressure of transforming into what I was destined to be. I just became—and that was a beautiful offering from my family.

Now more than ever, I see the gift in realizing that so many different and diverse people have grown up with me. So many people stand alongside me at work. Starting in the living room up until now. The growth is all exciting and interesting. It never gets old—when you're walking in your purpose, this is almost always the case. The journey is constantly beautiful and challenging.

Many things keep shifting in the relationship I have with my family. My mom was a kid having kids. So when I came of age, I decided that I would be the man of the house, and my purpose took on a new role. Be the provider that my mom never had. My dad was incarcerated most of my childhood. Therefore, I didn't have consistent examples of what it meant to be a man. Along the way, I learned on my own how to define manhood. Everything I do is a reflection of my family, and family is everything to me. It comes before my celebrity or any outward projections that the world may want for Omarion. To my family, I am Omari. As I grow closer to who I am, the dynamic of my family evolves.

I think it always will. I think that's what is so beautiful about having a close-knit family. We all take turns being a type of example for one another. I am the first one in my family to transform into who I am today as a person. Because of who I am, professionally, I can help people, which also feeds my destiny and gives drive to my purpose. No one knew this was going to happen. My aim continues to grow with my family because I'm the firstborn. My Nana taught me a lot about who I am and my family. She set the tone for almost everything I know. As she grows older, my brother, my cousins, and I are taking on more responsibility. We're keeping the family together like Nana taught us how. From organizing family functions and get-togethers to planning family events, we are stepping into our positions and contributing to the family as a whole. We're also developing a more profound understanding of what it means for us to keep our family intact.

When I was young in my career, these tasks weren't on my mind. I wanted to go hard for myself early on, but in hindsight, it was to go hard for my family, especially my kids. I wasn't thinking about seeing or spending time with Nana in this way. Time and age have changed that completely. And since having kids, I've become even more in tune with how vital legacy and purpose are. As a young rising star, I wasn't thinking about taking my kids to see their Nana. Those responsibilities didn't exist. I love this new life and a new way of moving through the world. I enjoy it because you get what you give to people and what you want to get in return. I have the energy and awareness now to put that intentional energy forward. It feels good, and I see that it helps. It supports my family, our health, and our commitment to each other. We all influence each other in such a positive way. So my purpose continues to grow with more responsibility and more information—it's really cool and such an honor.

Purpose starts with the intention to take on the task at hand. Uncovering the why of the passion we hold for something is vital. Once you figure out why you're doing something, you can discover and color in the rest. But I think that it's crucial that you're intentional. Sometimes people get hung up on that word, but our intentions don't have to be deep. We can set intentions for the most simple tasks like going to the grocery store to buy healthy ingredients to make a purposeful meal. Or we can create intentions around waking up early, before our work starts, to do that passion project we've been dreaming about.

Purpose and intention go hand in hand. They feed each other and make us more mindful about what we want to set out to do—how we want to live our lives. We want a particular outcome, but we can become distracted and confused if we don't set the tone for getting there. At the end of the day, purpose requires looking at all the moving parts in front of us. The impact you have starts with building confidence and being consistent. If you do something long enough or put yourself on a schedule, you will transform and get better. It doesn't matter what you do, you could do anything. If you do it over and over and over again, you'll get good at it. Certain things you have to stick with for a really long time to get good at. Dedication is necessary. That's where patience kicks in and fuels both the intentions set and the purpose that's driving you.

Don't get discouraged if you feel like you're at something for a long time. Time builds empires. When I look at my career, I see longevity in all facets. My purpose is the foundation that's carried me all these years. I've stood on this way of thinking for as long as I can remember. Throughout all my transitions, through all my peaks and valleys, I am still steady. Standing on my intention to keep being great, grounded, and filled with gratitude for the journey has supported my purpose.

Just because I live an intentional life aligned with my purpose in no way means I don't get tripped up by life. The goal is to always get back up anytime I fall. There were many times in my career where I thought, *Okay—is this it?* In those moments, I reminded myself that anything could happen and change. Dealing with record labels is tricky. If the label decides to support and invest in you, your experience could be fantastic. If not, that's a whole new story that isn't favorable most of the time. Being signed can make or break a career. It's an interesting game to be in. When there were moments of doubt for me, I had to shift my purpose as I knew it for the better. I've had to transform and continue growing with time.

When I sit down and think about how far I've come in my career, I am reminded that when you put your art into the Universe, it talks back to you—it sticks to people. As an artist, I've become etched into the lives of so many people. I regularly think about that conversation with the fan who had lost her friend. I remember the feeling I felt in my heart when she shared that he was buried with my photo. That experience, alongside the eye-opening trip to Australia, showed me that no matter what, no one can take your art from you. There is someone out there who needs to hear what you have to say, who wants to see what you have to offer, and whose life will be forever changed by it. So when in doubt, I'm reminded that my purpose doesn't just affect me. It's far-reaching and continuously evolving. Standing in my purpose, and realizing it, also shows me that life is not easy. It demonstrates that happiness is a choice, and in my work as a musician, it's my job to remind people of what joy embodies through the highs and lows. No matter what I've walked through, music creates community and brings us all together. Purpose is the language that's taught me that you will have to leave things behind and that everyone cannot and will not grow with you. It's taught me how to be resilient and relentless. Life is the longest shortest time, and with that, we should strive to do and be our best even in the face of fear, failure, and finding forever. When you're living your purpose, everything that presents itself is a lesson. We are multifaceted, and it's up to us to see ourselves and what we offer the world as valuable. If you're paying attention to your *why* in life, everything else will unfold in front of you. The stars will align wherever you are.

Ho'oponopono

An ancient Hawaiian Prayer on Forgiveness:

> I am sorry.
> Please forgive me.
> Thank you.
> I love you.

WHAT IT MEANS TO ME: I've used this mantra many times in my personal life and continue to hold it close. It reminds me to extend forgiveness to others and myself. It keeps me grounded in gratitude and respect for those around me, even when conflicts arise. This prayer mantra also holds me accountable when I am wrong and makes room for the acknowledgment of the pain I may have caused others. Speaking these words can help heal your karmic imprint and facilitate the necessary healing to move forward.

READER REFLECTION: Think of a moment in your life when you dropped the ball or made a mistake. Write it down or record it on your phone. Then meet it with the forgiveness prayer at the close of your writing or recording.

Affirmations for Success

Read these out loud in a seated position.

I am successful.

I can create the life I want.

I will work hard to change and grow.

I will devote myself to manifesting my dreams daily.

WHAT IT MEANS TO ME: Success looks and feels different for everyone. When it comes to my success, I don't equate it with what I have materially but what I have spiritually. I am a sacred being, and recognizing that, to me, is success. So often we can get stuck on thinking cars, money, notoriety, and extravagant things make us successful. Over the years, I have learned that is false. This affirmation for success is a reminder that we get to create the life we want on all different levels. What is successful to me may not be successful to you, and that is okay.

READER REFLECTION: Write in a journal a list of things that you want in your life and circle the things that you feel will make you feel successful and spiritually rich. Add to this list as often as you need to. Allow it to serve as a reminder that you are in charge of what success looks like in your life.

| PURPOSE MEDITATION |

I upload well-being and fulfillment into my heart's drive.
I upload my divine desire to stay connected to the source above.

I breathe.

I'm fulfilled each day by unlocking a new pathway to the source of inspiration.
When engaged in my purpose, life becomes easier and less complicated.

Well-being and wholeness build inner wealth.

Your mind is the true lasting source of happiness.

I breathe.

I give myself permission to enhance self-esteem and increase self-confidence so that I can fearlessly face difficulties and challenges.

I breathe.

I upload well-being and fulfillment into my heart's drive.
I upload my divine desire to stay connected to the source above.

I breathe.

Affirmations for Certainty

Read these out loud in a seated position.

I can hold my own.

I will choose to be the best version of myself.

I am worthy of everything good that comes my way.

I can choose where I want my focus to go.

I will accept things as they are.

I am valuable and no one can take that away from me.

WHAT IT MEANS TO ME: Clarity opens the door for self-doubt to leave. I am a big believer in being clear and confident as we navigate our relationships and the world around us. Confidently holding my own has shown me that I am worthy of everything good that comes my way. I can and will choose where I want my focus and energy to go. Acceptance is a part of my process. Trusting that I am valuable and that I bring something beneficial to the spaces I occupy reminds me that I am the master of my life.

READER REFLECTION: What are you sure and clear about in your life? Think about what you'd like to master in your life to live free and in alignment with your highest self. Write a list of these things in your journal.

2

Fear

Being afraid of something doesn't make you weak. It means you're human and capable of feeling all the feelings that come along with being a soul in a body. When I look at what activates my fear response, it's usually things I don't fully understand. At times we will fear what we don't know and what we can't control. But like I tell my daughter when she's afraid of the dark, just because you can't see it, doesn't mean you have to fear it. If we allow it, fear can be paralyzing. So much so that we do our best to avoid the things that blind us from seeing the truth behind the fear. I believe that turning toward the moments in life that make us want to flee is where we find a more in-depth understanding of ourselves, purpose, and the ability to expand. Welcoming what may be intimidating makes room in our life for practicing self-control and acceptance. I often tell my children that fear is an illusion and with that comes an opportunity for growth and a spirit of inquiry: *Why is this frightening? How can I make this productive instead of being paralyzed by the unknown?* As I learn more about myself and others, it's clear that the information on the other side of fear is more important than the fear itself. Trusting this, I've found a deeper sense of confidence and strength.

Affirmations for Fear

Read these out loud in a seated position.

This feeling will pass.

I am capable of moving through this.

My fear can teach me something.

I am a being of love and strength.

WHAT IT MEANS TO ME: I believe that words mean things. They can carry us through or break us down. Hope we speak to ourselves can be the deciding factor in how we go about our days and lives. Positive affirmations remind me that I am in control of my life and that I have the power and ability to live prosperously. Remembering my power is sacred makes room for me to grow when I forget my potential. We all have off days, and we have to remember to count on ourselves to be a nourishing source of support.

READER REFLECTION: What positive "I am" statements can you say out loud that will help you feel good about yourself and better throughout your day? Write them down and keep them where you can easily see them. Whenever you need a pick-me-up, read your affirmations out loud and remember who you are and who you want to be.

As I've grown in my career, one of the most significant take-aways I've kept close is that fear can not only stop us in our tracks but also cause us to stay there. Being stagnant isn't an option for me, because fear breeds laziness if you allow it. Laziness is a grave where brilliant ideas die. Give yourself permission to kill procrastination with action. Letting fear get in the way of the end goal doesn't serve us in the long run. It's easier to quit than it is to press forward. We cannot grow if our minds are operating in a paralyzed state. Being emotionally flexible, even when I've been apprehensive, is where I find my absolute power. The only thing we can do when greeted with fear is to face it—that will push us closer to our purpose and prepare us for abundance and perseverance. My inner voice reminds me to question the things I'm fearful of. It's in the moments of self-reflection when I ask myself, *Why won't you do that? Why are you hesitating?* Standing up for yourself in your journey is vital. If you allow it, fear will trick you out of trying. Life requires us to find solutions and remedies that work in tandem with our mission to become our best selves. If we quit because something scares us, that will be the ultimate defeat. Pressing forward through fear and uncertainty can motivate us in new ways and encourage an authentic relationship with the things that we struggle with the most. This has helped me articulate my position in life—and it also helps me figure out what obstacles are trying to teach me. More often than not, we are in our own way. I've been there. Digging deep and being honest with ourselves is a key component of the self-awareness we're born to unlock. In this life, we are never without a test even if that test is facing ourselves and trusting that we can make a way out of no way.

When I first got into the music industry, I was signed to a record label. I was sixteen years old and had a deal with Sony Epic Records. Before we got signed as B2K, I clearly remember going to audition for L.A. Reid. LaFace Records represented some really hot artists at that time, from Pink to Usher. We had seen major labels already, all of whom passed on signing us, but this was one we admired and felt connected to. So when we got the call to get on a plane and go to Atlanta for the first time, we knew for sure we were about to be signed. We rehearsed our dance moves and showcased performance tirelessly waiting for our moment. In our minds, the deal was done. This wasn't our first showcase, we were ready, and we brought our confidence to the room as always. Nothing scared us; we were fearless and ready to show up. If practice makes perfect, we were damn near perfect. Our game faces were on, and we went to that audition to shut shit down. We were ready to secure what we *knew* was meant for us.

LaFace Records passed on us. It was disappointing, but we knew giving up wasn't an option. We had to keep going—so we did. Up until that point, none of the labels knew what to do with us. In that era of the new millennium, there were no black boy groups like B2K. There wasn't a formula for us. We were different on every level and required an entirely new blueprint. Having a label that was excited for us to represent their company in the music business was a key to our success. We needed people to believe in us just as much as we believed in ourselves. Over the years, I learned the importance of patience and paying attention to what matters most. As a performer, there's a lot of waiting and preparation before the seeds we sow start taking root and bearing fruit. Being turned down by LaFace Records after being turned down by so many others before was a test of patience and, ultimately, perseverance.

There was one more record company to see, Sony Epic Records. This was our last chance to get a deal. Management shared with our parents that the Sony Epic showcase would be the last before moving on from the group. It was made clear that if Sony didn't sign us, that would be the end of the road. The pressure was on. We had to get this deal—there was no other option. The guys and I ended up performing at the Sony Los Angeles office, and that audition ended up being the one to send us to New York for yet another showcase.

Polly Anthony, Dave Mcpherson, Max Gousse, and so many other important people were in attendance. We had on our superstar uniforms, denim from head to toe. We were ready to give it all we had—and we did—we got the deal! This was our moment, but the work was far from over.

Preparing for our debut album was thrilling. Life was moving so fast, and we were so young, eager to entertain. We recorded in big cities known for being interwoven within the heart of music. We traveled to places like New York and Atlanta to record with Tricky Stewart, The-Dream, and other iconic producers for our breakout hit and self-titled album. B2K was embarking on boy band history. We were ready to take over the world and be the absolute best to ever do it. I learned a lot about being an individual in a group during this time. The biggest takeaway highlights the beauty of togetherness even when operating individually. I learned so much about my distinctiveness in B2K. Wherever I go, even all these years later, I remember that no matter where I am or whom I'm with, I have to stay committed to being my true self.

IF YOU DON'T HAVE A
DESTINATION, YOU
CAN REALLY GET LOST.
PAY ATTENTION TO
YOUR ENVIRONMENT,
ENERGY, AND PATH.

When I transitioned to being a solo artist, the music business was changing in big ways around that time. My album *21* debuted at number one on the US Billboard charts, selling over one hundred thousand copies in its first week. I finally started to feel like I was aligned with my work and surrounded by people who truly wanted the best for me. Donnie Ienner, Lisa Ellis, and Kawan Prather were invested in my success on a new level. They believed in my growth as an artist. But then everyone I had been working with and who was in my corner started leaving or getting fired. It felt like my champions were dwindling, one by one. I couldn't help but be a little afraid about what the future held for me. I had a hit album with *21*, but the next steps were hazy, since the people who helped make it happen were leaving the label. I reminded myself that I was built for this. I had grown to know patience and trust extremely well—and still the unknown felt intimidating.

With everyone leaving, I knew that I needed to get out of that deal. Everything I worked so hard for was in jeopardy. Going independent felt like the next thing to explore. Embarking on my independence was exciting and gave me more responsibility for my craft. And though I didn't know what was next, moving forward into this chapter of my life was necessary and unavoidable. I couldn't let the fear of the unknown stop me from creating my legacy. So even through the fog of not knowing, I still felt like there was something designed just for me and within my control as an artist and entertainer.

| Energy Check: Fear

What's your earliest memory of fear?

What was your parents' relationship with fear?

Do you fear change?

Are you willing to overcome your fears to accomplish something great?

Do you fear the truth?

Failure comes with success. We have to do both, at some point, to know what they feel like. Just like we can't truly know joy if we aren't acquainted with pain. Being scared to fail shrinks our ability to fully live and truly love. If you're too scared to try, you'll stay stuck and unable to move forward and level up. What I am continually learning on my journey is that I can use fear to charge myself up. And it allows me to access my highest self despite not knowing what's next. When I was a kid, I remember the fearlessness I had. I taught myself how to backflip at a very young age—off fences, park benches, cars, you name it, without any hesitation or care in the world. I just did it. There are moments in my adulthood when I realize I'm not *that* kid anymore. My maturity as a man, and role as a father, makes me more aware of the risks that come with being fearless.

Now more than ever, both personally and professionally, I find myself facing fear in new ways—and looking at it through a different lens. For example, I used to obsess over the outcome of certain situations, and now I realize and accept that things will be how they will be. There's no use obsessing over what cannot be changed. And acceptance has taught me that you can always dust yourself off and try again. Not being scared of the outcomes allows me to be fully present and in the moment. Learning something new can be terrifying. You don't know what to expect. Fear can either make you back down or encourage you to face your obstacles head-on.

What I've realized is that in order for me to have an impact through my work, I have to exercise my ability to push through and show up no matter what's standing in front of me. It's in these moments that I'm reminded of the bravery I had as a kid doing flips and tricks off anything I could. Resilience is born from the moments that frighten us. There is power in being flexible with our fears and trusting that a lesson can emerge through it. My experiences have had a profound effect on me, and one thing that I realized is what I want to accomplish in business. I had to step back and realize the kinds of players that I was on the team with, that there's a good side and a bad side. The good side is that I could maintain my joy and relationship with my creativity as an artist. Many people don't realize that if your life isn't going well, it's tough to create. Creativity will escape us when we aren't happy with ourselves in life. I've always maintained a level of clarity and a great relationship with creativity. It's covered me throughout my whole experience. It had so much of an effect on me that, you know, my business was being neglected. That was the wrong aspect of it, and it taught me a lot about starting where I was when it was time to learn to do things differently.

I was working and being represented by people who I thought had my best interest at heart, but they didn't. I had to step back and realize what kind of work was ahead when I embarked on my own. I had to think a lot about what kinds of people would represent me and my vision going forward. Learning the hard way helped mold where I am today with my brand. I've figured out how to be all-encompassing—as a man, as a creative, as a human being—who has this unique life experience and who is dedicated to contributing to the world. My goal in life is to create joy for myself and my family. It's been imperative with all my experiences that I've been able to step back and recognize what a great support system looks like. And what it means to be surrounded by people who aren't just doing things for their own best interest. We are all a part of this shared experience. It's so much more beneficial to keep yourself and others in mind. This is a far-reaching benefit. It creates a better place for a beautiful experience.

EVERY DECISION THAT WE MAKE IN LIFE IS LINKED TO AN OUTCOME.

The greatest lesson fear has presented to me is the ability to confront and question its presence in my life. There are certain experiences that I had to let go of to move past the hesitancy of beginning again. Learning how to start from scratch required me to let go of my old ways and reintroduce myself to a better way of living, eating, and being physically active. While this may seem to be a mundane example, learning to release the unhealthy habits I picked up, so that I could relearn new ones, took bravery, dedication, and commitment to pursuing the unknown, which can feel daunting to anyone. When we conquer our fears, valuable information is displayed that helps us become more confident in who we are and what we're called to do in life.

I am also constantly mindful to not allow my fear to guide my footsteps but instead to let it lead the way to a deeper understanding of myself and my experiences—past and present—and the endless possibilities that stand before me when I show up bravely. If I let fear become a distraction, I will miss out on opportunities to grow. Growth is always the goal. If we can find the courage to greet our fear as a teacher, we can shift our perspective. We can then take what we learn and support other people on their journey to becoming their best. My highest self emerges to take on any challenge that fear presents. Because I didn't have anyone walking me into this knowledge, the best knowledge I could get was my experience.

In learning along that way, I found out how to identify the missing pieces in my life. That's a wonderful thing, and it's gotten me to this point now. If you can see enough to get the lesson, you can continue being happy in your experience. So many things in life are situational. But they're also preparing us for the next level or higher growth. Even with everything I've gone through in my life, I never allow anybody to rattle my cage. During my process, I've stayed confident in my work. Nothing can convince me that my work is not purposeful. My greatest lessons come from not quitting and always believing in the possibility of evolving.

If you're prepared for everything, nothing can surprise you. Do your due diligence and make sure you understand your commitments contractually. Learn every aspect of your business and make it a point to know. Trust the process. Doubt and fear kill dreams and courage. Trust your gut. In times of feeling uncertain, I remembered all that I've already accomplished in life. The goal isn't to do things perfectly; it's to grow and expand what you're capable of. This is the key to not letting fear dominate our thoughts and actions. It's a marathon, not a sprint, and I will continue to pace myself.

Growing can be rewarding and painful at the same time— but this is the magic of emotions and the very fabric of great art. I have found that there is a fear paradox: fear fuels my ability to be fearless. It's almost like a friendship of sorts. One that holds me accountable and requires my hard work and effort. Having a past is what creates history. What is meant for you and your life, no one can have or take away. I've always been proud of everything that I've done creatively. Rarely do I think twice about presenting my art to people. This is what I was born to do. I believe that with all my heart. I have great confidence in what I do, which I think sets me apart from many people. I don't second-guess myself, and I'm not scared of showing up as my whole self. Sharing my craft, even in such a dog-eat-dog industry, hasn't instilled much fear in me. Still, it has made me more curious about perfecting my art. Such is the fear paradox: when thinking about fear, I think about fearlessness. I'm excited by things I know little about. My relationship with fear is healthy and has to be entertained because that is how I learn, grow, and become better.

As I think about fear and how it leads me to deeper curiosity, I am reminded that it's a mirror. It's confirmation within our own selves to be open to whatever shows up at our door. Some days I feel like it's a constant attraction to becoming my higher self. What I've learned over the years is to question everything. If I make a decision, what will happen? I think we all need to be more serious about this—about teaching ourselves how to face fear and press forward. I didn't grow up with meaningful examples or male role models on how to do this.

From a young age, I had to move through the world as my own teacher. fending for myself so learning on my own became second nature. I became extremely confident and grew comfortable with curiosity. To this day, I believe on a granular level that the things that call me are meant for me. Whatever arrives at my door is a teacher, and I am always open to learning. I am constantly asking myself, where am I being led and why? I don't turn away from fear because I know there is a lesson, something I can take away from moments of anxiety or uncertainty. I have to credit my mom for giving me the space to explore things. I don't turn away from fear because I know there is a lesson, something I can take away from moments of anxiety or uncertainty. I have to credit my mom for giving me the space to explore things. Having the freedom to explore the world around me so freely built a relationship with fear that made me fearless. My mom instilled in me that there was nothing I couldn't do. That set the tone for bravery and perseverance in my childhood. I believe fearlessness stems from the confidence that parents display. My mom is the most fearless person I know. She led by example, and that translated into how I move through the world. So even without a father figure, I felt prepared for the world and the experiences I would encounter. To this day, there's not much that I'm scared of or think that I can't handle.

I'm always ready to take the risk and ask hard questions to uncover my *why*. It's in that discovery that my curiosity leads me to the many lessons of life. Sometimes we all have to find out the hard way. I've encountered the good, the bad, the different, and the challenging. I've seen that being curious is really what you make it. Suppose you pay close attention to all that is presenting itself, and you have the ability to befriend awareness. You'll be able to see who you are and why you're connected with the things around you. Our life and the obstacles that rear their head are reflections of what we need to learn. They remind us where we need to grow and become better. Being scared of that won't change the truth. Being curious will deepen our inner wisdom and remind us of our divine power.

Not having a male role model to teach me how to be a man wasn't an excuse for me not to show up and do the work in my life. I refused to make it one. I became the role model I didn't have. At a certain point, I had to find the courage and look at my life. Even if I did have a father figure or a mentor, I would have still had to decipher what lessons to keep or discard. I would have had to learn what it meant to stand on my own, face my fears, and uncover my truths. I was willing, even without guidance, to accept what called me. It was my responsibility to listen to what the Universe was presenting to me. Everything we come up against in life, no matter our circumstances, can be a reflection of who we are.

Being honest with ourselves will change the game and the healing at hand. Curiosity can and will educate you. It has taught me how to get to know myself on a deeper level in my personal life. When I've been faced with moments of fear, I've also discovered moments of clarity. This is how I learned many lessons through life, even without someone leading the way.

There will be moments when we are all we have. Some of us grow to understand this earlier than others. Some of us are meant to learn alone. It's in that solitude and solo exploration that we find our true selves. We all, at some point in our lives, have to do something for ourselves as an individual and as human beings. We won't always be inspired or led by someone else. Many paths will require us to journey without a guide but with self-trust and belief in hand. This takeaway has made me feel whole and brave. It's taught me that in fear, there is fearlessness. I value the world and its lessons in a big way because of the gift of knowledge. Fear has taught me how to be brave and how to step into my power.

Om

A sacred Hindu + Tibetan Hinduism symbol
Sound: 432hz frequency – AUM

WHAT IT MEANS TO ME: As a musician, the frequency of chanting Om, a sacred sound in Hinduism and Tibetan Buddhism, elevates my understanding on a deeper level and brings me closer to the present moment of being alive. It reminds me that my body is a tool and a source of divine power. Om (or Aum) is said to signify the spirit of ultimate reality and consciousness. Om is traditionally used at the start and finish of meditation and is known to some as the original sound of the universe. This deeply powerful vibration (432Hz) plays an important role in the cycle of life, and it supports me in recentering during my meditation practice. Om is a syllable that can be chanted individually or in a group. Its vibration is grounding and cleansing to the mind, body, and spirit—it's something you can tangibly feel; it's not just a word. It's an action.

READER REFLECTION: Take a moment to pause and breathe. Drop your shoulders, unclench your jaw, close your eyes, or focus on something in front of you. When you feel ready, take a deep breath in. On the exhale, release the sound Om until you can't any longer. Tune in to your body before and after this practice. Take note of how you feel at the start, and how you feel at the end. Write it down, reflect, and find space in your daily life for this sacred and grounding practice.

FEAR MEDITATION

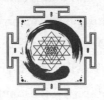

I am not perfect.

I celebrate my patience.

I gain strength, courage, and confidence when I face my fears.

I respond thoughtfully to negativity—I do not react.

I breathe.

I am open to greater possibilities.

I become stronger in the face of doubt.

I can overcome anxiety and fear by controlling my breathing.

I breathe.

I trust that my choices grant me peace.

I am open to the changes that will greet me on this path.

I accept the lessons and the divine timing.

I breathe.

Affirmations for Strength

Read these out loud in a seated position.

My mind is sound and strong.

My heart is open and filled with love.

My body is working in my favor.

My inner strength is abundant.

I am mentally and physically strong.

WHAT IT MEANS TO ME: Trusting my inner strength reminds me to stand in my power. It's an invitation to keep my mind sound and strong. These words are pillars to my life. I am constantly reminded that my body is working in my favor and in harmony with my inner strength. It's important for me to keep in mind that I am mentally and physically strong, even through moments of adversity.

READER REFLECTION: List your strengths in your journal and reread them daily. Positive affirmation is essential, and this will serve as a reminder to not doubt how resilient and capable you are.

Five Acts of Joy (self-expression)

As you read through this book, I want you to think about your five acts of joy. Below are some practices that I deeply resonate with. They keep me grounded and remind me to come back to the center when I'm feeling off. As an entertainer, father, and businessman, it can be easy to get thrown off track. I have a lot on my plate, so I must stay intentional about reconnecting with my joy, my body, and my energetic practices. It's important that we all carve out the time to get in touch with ourselves and our happiness.

Making sure that I stay rooted and in touch with myself is not only a daily practice but a spiritual one. Being a man of color and a single father, it's essential to actively take care of myself and intentionally tap into what I need. I am grateful that my breath and movement are free. There are so many people in the world who cannot say the same. Making music, singing, and journaling are reminders of my power to access my true and highest self. All of these acts of joy make room for me to be deeply curious about my life, myself, and the imprint I am leaving behind. I'd like to encourage you to tap into the things and practices that allow you to feel fully and truly connected to yourself and your bliss. This is your permission to get curious about everything you may have been putting aside or avoiding. Joy is our birthright. Rest and recalibration are too. The goal is to create a list of things that also allows you to create consistency and spiritual accessibility in your life. No one can do this hard work for us. It is up to us, and us alone, to name the things that give us the freedom to self-reflect, self-express, and self-correct.

BREATHWORK. Breath is life. In intense moments, breathing helps me take the necessary steps to recenter, calm down, and bring awareness back to my body. As an artist, it reminds me to expand, release, and project. Intentional breathing also allows me to access more positive energy through laughter and to be mindful about the peaks and valleys in my life.

MOVEMENT. Having a relationship with music reminds me to find joy in dance and body movement. From being in the studio to the gym to riding my bike—being in motion shapes gratitude in my life and makes room for me to let go and be in tune with the moment.

SINGING. Singing is praise. In my life, it's a joyful expression that allows me to emotionally share myself and my energy. Words have power, and music activates energy in those who listen. It is the universal language of togetherness.

WRITING. Writing acts as a mirror in my life. It allows me to be in touch with myself—no matter what I am going through. I use it as a way to express my thoughts and feelings and to reflect.

PIANO. This instrument is therapeutic for me and inspires me to focus. I didn't think I would grow to have such a close relationship with the piano—but it serves as a place of peace for me. Playing reminds me that there is joy through music without words.

| Energy Check: Journal Prompts

Make a list of your five acts of joy.

Reflect on how you can practice daily joy in your life.

3

Manhood

Every real man should have a grip on his ability to focus. We have to learn to be in a place where creating our reality and standing in our truth is learned even when we don't have an example to follow. I know that may seem counterintuitive or even easier said than done. But I believe we all have a choice to create the life we want and to be the person we may have needed growing up. It all comes down to betting on yourself, trusting the path you're on, and recognizing when the table has been set for you. Growing up in a single-parent household with my mom, I had to learn how to be a man in an unconventional way. Early on, I adopted the man of the house role. My father was incarcerated, and his absence shaped me. I remember longing for a role model to look up to and learn from.

Back then, I didn't know his absence was shaping me to grow into a more compassionate and loving person. It wasn't until my dad and I reconnected in adulthood that I understood just how sacred forgiveness was for self-liberation and empathetic understanding was for personal growth. Something extremely admirable about my father was his ability to take responsibility for his shortcomings as a parent. When we reconnected years after I had grown up, we didn't need to rehash what the truth was; we both knew it. We did, however, grow to have a better understanding for each other and our individual paths. I don't blame him for doing what he didn't know how to do. My parents were teenagers when they had me. My dad was fifteen and my mother was sixteen. There was so much learning they had to do when I was born. They were kids. My dad lacked the tools and resources to show up for me the way I needed him to. If he had the tools, I can honestly say that our experience together as father and son would have been very different. But even in my dad's absence, I learned that the only thing I could control was myself. Being overly focused on what I didn't have wouldn't change anything. The only thing that truly mattered was choosing to be present in my life and make healthier choices, mentally, emotionally, and physically, as I grew into a man. It's not only what you say that matters: it's also how you actively show up in the world.

In reconnecting with my dad, his actions spoke louder than anything he could ever say. He was committed to getting to know me and doing right by me, even though we had lost years. As we started to rebuild our relationship, it made me reflect on how I was committed to healing moving forward. Yes, I had been disappointed growing up. Yes, I felt like I was lacking and missing a piece of myself. I yearned for that kind of relationship between myself and a male role model. But even in my feelings of confusion or lack around not having a male figure in my life, I was being given a new chance to flex my growth muscle and show up as the man my mother raised me to be. This new journey into manhood was illuminating. Not taking things personally, even when it was very hard not to, has carried me through life. It's also allowed me to accept people and all their human complexities with less judgment and more love.

Learning how to be a man on my own consisted of many pivotal moments. There are things that I learned the hard way, simply because I didn't know which way to go. Trial and error presented itself a lot to me, and being a student of life very quickly showed me the things I needed to change about myself for myself. Not having a father figure to teach me how to communicate as a man, or what to watch for, or how to treat women made it clear to me that I needed to take responsibility for myself and my actions sooner rather than later. It was easy to float around ignorant in my early years, but as I grew spiritually and emotionally, I had to be the man I'd been missing for myself.

My mom being the grounded woman that she is always made sure that I knew I had a choice. This was one of those choices. To show up and do the hard thing: change and grow into my best self. No excuses. My mom always made sure I knew that I could be who I wanted to be in this life—but I'd have to work for it. I think of all the times she would take me and my brother, O'Ryan, to the hair salon where she would work long hours. Watching her work and create the best life she could for us was incredibly inspiring. There was no fussing or complaining, she just showed up. While she couldn't teach me the ins and outs of how to be a man, she showed me through her work ethic, loving support, and kind spirit that I am in charge of my destiny regardless of my circumstances. My mom reminded me of my purpose whenever I swayed. She's the reason I dance and sing and have the career that I have. She stressed to my siblings and I that we could create the lives we wanted. And if she could make a way raising me and my siblings, well before age thirty, then I had no excuses.

Even in moments of confusion or uncertainty, I remembered her wisdom and could recall her actions. Both showed me clearly that I would never be lacking if I've made a home within myself. My mom never settled. She showed me through her dedication and grit that nothing would be handed to us. Showing up and taking care of your business was not only a method of survival but a testament to integrity and character. I took these lessons with me as I grew up and became a man and father. Everything I learned by way of how I was raised and how I experienced the world gave me some great insight on how to move through my challenges and success in my personal and professional life. I believe that higher power, spirit guides, and ancestors were leading the way for me. I was open to every lesson even if it was hard to grasp at first. Finding my way by myself shaped me into a man of resilience with a divine belief that I was chosen to be on the planet for a reason. At a young age, I knew that I had to step it up. I don't recall feeling intimidated by this. But I do remember feelings of being shocked by some of the things I had to walk through.

| Energy Check: Manhood

What is divine masculinity?

How important is it for a man to stand on his word?

How important is it for a man to show a boy what he will become one day?

What are things worth protecting as a man?

What is essential for a man to understand about a woman?

Once I got in B2K and started really doing my thing, I left a lot of stuff behind. A shedding was happening. My relationships were changing and shifting, and without realizing it I became increasingly distant from my family when I left home to pursue my career. I just thought it was normal. My saving grace during that period, when I wasn't as present or intentional as I am now, was a simple fact that lessons kept coming up repeatedly. It wasn't until I started paying attention that I realized that being a man was up to me. I had to make my own way and set my own tone for the life I wanted to have and experience.

I embarked on my own personal journey for a higher purpose—to learn who I was as an individual outside my family unit. I had to do this at a very young age, which boosted my maturity and taught me how to be deliberate in my actions. My grounding foundation started at this point. Leaving my family to embark on this new journey of professionalism and manhood allowed us to grow. I was going out into the world in this new and big way, but my family was not. I knew then that I was the man of the house and that I had a job to do. When I would come back home from touring and performing, I could see and feel the difference in myself and my family. Changes were happening, and I was learning how to be the man I wanted to be. I was dedicated to my future and knew that I had to stay committed and determined.

Something that kept me going was being able to call upon my family whenever needed. My family was my rock, and I was theirs. Even as I was navigating manhood and the many lessons I was learning along the way, my mom always believed in me and supported me no matter what. To me, that's value. Support is valuable. I was so happy to experience that throughout my life—because people really get lost inside the fast-paced motion of success. I have a level of determination, focus, and persistence. I've been this way my whole life. Any and everything that I've ever put my mind to, I've always succeeded at. Nothing can throw me off. Being myself and realizing and recognizing that the outside world can't shake me allowed me to stay clear and aligned with the greater good.

When I became a member of B2K, I was the last person to join. Being the fourth member showed me a lot about the importance of individuality. It's easy to get lost if you're not sure of yourself. In the beginning, I thought we were forming a brotherhood, but it became increasingly clear that that was not the case. There were many times in the lifetime of B2K that made me feel like I didn't belong and that I was replaceable. We were kids still learning and growing and trying to figure out who we truly were. The bumping heads, the jealousy, being mismanaged, and everything else in between showed me that it was time to elevate myself and really step into being the artist that I was committed to being.

Separating from the group opened up a whole new set of lessons that I needed to learn. Sometimes you have to revisit old chapters to really grow from them. After going solo, I remember thinking that I wished it was easier to just leave that old chapter in the past. Yet I could not seem to shake the connection. Everywhere I went, I was reminded that B2K would be embedded in my identity forever. I was pretty frustrated because I didn't understand why B2K overshadowed me as a solo artist and would never go away. My career had shown that I was more successful on my own. I looked to people in the industry and compared our careers as group artists—like Beyoncé, Justin Timberlake, and even Michael Jackson. They've been able to completely break free of their group being so heavily tied to who they were. I felt like there was always something reminding me that I was a part of B2K, even when I wasn't anymore. I couldn't grasp what that was about. Perhaps I needed to change my mindset and see if there was a lesson I was missing.

Before committing to the Millennium Tour, JBoog wanted to have a phone call. We hadn't spoken in years prior to the reuniting being back on the table. I was hesitant to be on the road with them because we didn't end on good terms, to say the least. There was a huge public fallout where my character and integrity were attacked on public radio. I found out on Power 106 that the other band members planned to replace me. As you can imagine, that was a shock and that shit pissed me off. I was being bashed and disrespected due to mismanagement, envy, and the elders around us who were instigating and causing further conflict. The tension was still thick from dealing with that. Everyone saw a brotherhood on the outside—this perfect boy band that was on top of the world—but behind the scenes, B2K was a tragedy. I had grown a lot since then, and truthfully, I wasn't sure I wanted to reconnect and go back to that place.

Despite my hesitancy to talk, I obliged, even though I didn't think there was much for either of us to say. My goal was to maintain professionalism at all times, especially after our rough history. This phone call really spoke to my growth, because I had a lot of conflicting feelings about everyone in the group, including Boog. Being dogged on the radio, in addition to the behind-the-scenes dysfunction, would have made it easy for me to want to fight versus talk things out. This phone call was an invitation to be a master of my mind and control my actions like I'd been practicing. Evolution in this instance looked like being the bigger person and not getting sucked into other people's bad character. Also, I believe in redemption and forgiveness, so I showed up and listened to what he had to say. I kept my composure and chose the higher road, which I've done at every turn in my career. It would have been easy to play the blame game and get caught up in things that didn't matter. Choosing to preserve and protect my energy from anything that could threaten it spoke volumes as to how far I had come.

The conversation went fine, and after our call, I had to sit and think about what the end goal was. There were many questions and feelings that went unanswered, but at the end of the day, I knew moving forward with the tour would not only make history but would shape me into an even better person, a person who has grown and changed a lot. Growth is something that is happening consistently and on so many different levels whether or not you choose it.

Deciding to reunite and go back on tour with the fellas was the most intense thing that I ever agreed to. I saw it as a challenge to myself. I had to learn how to compartmentalize in a way that I hadn't before. Rehearsals were tense. I felt like I was being tested from every angle. There were instances where I didn't want to move forward. What we need to do is not always what we want to do, but I knew that there was something important that could be gained by going back. When the tour went from idea to option to plan, it was time for me to trust my path. The table was set; it was time for me to show up and perform. It was like I was being injected back into a reality that I once created for myself. But this time I was coming back as a man; I had information and tools that I didn't have before.

One of my main takeaways during the tour was that being intentional and not letting anyone sway me from my focus held priority. It was step one in keeping my energy uplifted and positive. I've always been an optimistic person, but when I was a younger member of the group I didn't understand the importance of prioritizing groundedness. Yet on the Millennium Tour, fifteen years after B2K parted ways, things were different. I made the choice to be more aligned with my truth than anything else. That is what I had spent my adulthood cultivating—as a father, as a son, as an artist, as a businessman, as a man—and even in shitty situations, this was no different. I had to learn how to be grounded in the face of adversity and discomfort. Life teaches us that there is always something to be learned. Doing the tour was an olive branch and an opportunity for growth, and that shaped me.

| MANHOOD MEDITATION |

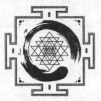

I am unlocking my authenticity.

I exercise self-control to stay in tune with my reality.

I am exceptional.

I engage in healthy and positive relationships.

I am flexible in my mindset.

I create an environment of growth and success.

I am grounded in truth.

I exercise courage and live in harmony with my ideas.

I am connected to my divine source.

I engage with my surroundings and purpose authentically.

I am dependable and truthful.

I fearlessly create the life that I want.

I am unlocking my authenticity.

I know now that we are all just echoes of our village realities. The women who ran my village did so with ethics and morals. And those morals that my mother and Nana instilled in me were to stay grounded in my truth and my word, which helped me navigate the reunion with B2K. All my life I've watched my Nana show up in her craft of making things and bringing her gift of creativity to the world. She's raised children and grandchildren and opened her home to those in need. Watching her nurture, love, and feed folks was pivotal for me to see. Her ability to be compassionate, creative, and steadfast at every turn is a stunning example of resilience and being committed to something greater than yourself. My mother has that same drive and love in her. I come from strong and loving women who don't just love their blood family; they love everyone.

That display of kindness, even when things aren't sweet in life or relationships, is what has helped me navigate everything like a man. Our village is what molds us. Whom we love and how we love are what shapes us. I know that everybody didn't have the gift of that experience. So when it was time for me to lead with forgiveness, compassion, and love, I had to bring the examples my mom and Nana left me with to the surface. Being reunited with B2K, I felt like I developed a superpower. The superpower was not letting anything or anyone lead me away from love with their poor behavior, past or present. Performing under this pressure and being able to truly focus and give all of my energy to the songs, I had to forget everything that we had been through and really be in the moment. There's something blissful about being able to let go—and that opportunity afforded me that. While I was prepared for anything, I knew that I needed to control my emotions and keep the goal priority: make history.

IT'S EASY TO GET LOST IF YOU'RE NOT SURE OF YOURSELF.

The process wasn't easy. The future is unknown. As I've matured, when instances happen that link the past with the present, it's important to remember that there's a moment for me to grow. Reflection on the past is something I did a lot during the tour. It would have been easy for me to get caught up in its negativity if I wasn't rooted in purpose and intention. I made a decision that I was going to finish what I started and see what the journey had in store for me. And I'm so happy that I did. It reinvigorated the light of my path. I felt like that path was getting dark for me, just in terms of the respect that I think I deserve. I realized that I had never seen the steps to how a man earns it. The answer: through hard work. As I continued to work hard, I began earning the respect of myself. Instead of looking externally, I looked internally and everything became so much clearer. True self-respect is so powerful and something that can never be taken away. I have a warrior mentality, and I will always fight for myself. I had business to handle, and it had to get done. However, the work isn't done. This was just one test of many in the course of manhood, but when I look back on it, I know that I aced that shit.

| Energy Check: Journal Prompts

Think about a pivotal moment in your life that encouraged you to change and walk in greater alignment with your purpose.

Make a list of the lessons you learned along the way.

What's been hard about your process?

Where has triumph shown up in your life after hardship?

How are you showing up to live the life you say you want to live?

IF YOU LET PEOPLE THROW YOU OFF, THEY WILL. YOU MUST MAINTAIN YOUR FOCUS.

GROWTH IS EVER PRESENT. MICRO CHANGES ARE HAPPENING AT EVERY TURN IN LIFE. CHANGING ALLOWS US TO LEAN INTO ACCEPTANCE. THERE IS SO MUCH IMPORTANCE IN CLARITY AND LEARNING WHAT AREAS IN LIFE NEED ATTENTION. IF GROWTH IS ALLOWED, CHANGE CAN HAPPEN IN OUR LIVES.

PART 2 |
PHYSICAL

4

Mastering Emotions: Unbothered

| MASTERING EMOTIONS MEDITATION |

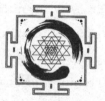

I can trust myself even when negativity greets me.

I breathe.

I will control myself for the best outcome.

I breathe.

I trust that my decisions direct me to my highest potential.

I breathe.

I belong in the presence and wholeness of peace.

I breathe.

I grow when I am self-aware and connected to my emotions.

I breathe.

I seek clarity through the knowledge of self.

I breathe.

I feel a sense of inner strength when I am open to vulnerability.

I breathe.

I am content and accepting of the present moment.

I breathe.

Embarking on the Millennium Tour was one of the most challenging moments in my career. Reconnecting with B2K after a messy breakup wasn't easy by any means. There was so much pressure to perform even when we weren't getting along. Tension filled the air so thick some days that you could literally feel it. But I had a job to do. And as a performer, I took my job very seriously. Everyone from the stage crew to the band, dancers, and sound techs were there because of us. They were counting on us to do our part so that they could do theirs and, in turn, take care of themselves and their families. There was no way that I could let the adversity I had been facing with the group get in the way of so many other moving parts. Choosing to show up and not be reactive to the negativity that could be a distraction was intentional. Mastering my emotions through a forty-four-date tour almost seemed like one of the most impossible things I could accomplish as a man.

Usually, people aren't finding themselves in a position like this—where they're back on tour with people who dragged them through the mud and infiltrated their personal life in a disrespectful way. No one chooses to go on tour with people they have tumultuous relationships with. In one breath, shit could pop off at any moment, but putting myself in this position was a pivotal moment for me and my growth. It was a beautiful moment, looking back on it today. The Millennium Tour was historic. We brought fans back to their childhoods: it was completely invigorating to look out into the crowd and see the people who grew up with B2K and our music be in such an amazing space of joy and nostalgia, despite what was going on behind the scenes. There was much power in learning more about being emotionally intelligent and deciding to stand in my power. Feeding into the negativity was not an option for me, no matter how hard it was not to.

I've been thinking a lot about what I would tell my children if they were in a similar situation as I was, and what I would teach them about moving through hardship. Life is hard. People will hurt us. And even with that being a part of the truth and a part of our human experience, we get to decide where our emotional energy goes. There is divinity in choosing not to be reactive when things get uncomfortable or when someone intentionally hurts us. Unforeseen occurrences happen all the time. I instill in them that they have the strength that it takes to know what to do. Outside of leading by example for my children, A'mei and Megaa, I do my best to communicate with them in a way that they can understand. I've had conversations with the two of them about how important it is to get curious about the adversity in front of them. As a grown man who had just walked through the tensions of a tour with former bandmates, in teaching my children to find curiosity in hard moments, I was also teaching myself.

JUST BECAUSE YOU'VE
HAD A FUCKED-UP
EXPERIENCE IN THE
PAST DOESN'T MEAN
YOU HAVE TO KEEP THAT
CYCLE GOING. CHOOSE
TO DO SOMETHING
DIFFERENT. CHOOSE TO
DO BETTER. CHOOSE
TO BE GREAT.

The world knows the very public humiliation connected with my children's mother and bandmate. Their relationship—and the overall tension and embarrassment—happened while I was on tour, which further pushed me into mastering how I responded and how I showed up—not only in my work but also in my personal life. Spiritually, a lot of things were shifting for me, and I refused to let the distraction of other people's inner turmoil bleed out onto me and throw me off my game. I could have fought with Fizz throughout the tour. I could have refused to co-parent with the mother of my children. I could have talked about this complicated family situation publicly to shame them. But I didn't. Reacting that way wouldn't have helped anything. I wasn't interested in dealing with them on that low vibrational level. I was being tested energetically—and I was committed to staying close to my integrity not only for me but also for my children. I knew they were watching me, more closely than I may have noticed.

My behavior during this emotionally trying time mattered. When we have children, they are paying close attention to us even when we don't think they are. If we aren't careful, our behaviors and shortcomings can re-create and manifest themselves in unhealthy ways to our offspring. Mastering my emotions showed me, first hand, that I was only in charge of myself. And how people saw me, especially during this tumultuous time, was important. How my kids see me, when they look back years later, and see the videos circulating online about this, is important.

How we show up and act in this world matters. And I also want my behavior to be a reflection of that in a good light. Of course, I'm not perfect, but I am committed to being honest, kind, and clear. That is vital for me and valuable for my children. As a person with freedom and autonomy, it's essential to know when to take a step forward and not get caught up in what you're leaving behind.

Knowing what kind of footprint you want to leave on this planet requires making deliberate choices even when the voyage tests your patience. My footprints are the stepping-stones for my kids—leading with love and compassion was my only option. I hope that A'mei and Megaa take away the importance of patience when they get older and eventually learn about this experience with me and their mother. I hope they gather wealth and knowledge about relationships and the value of taking time to know themselves and grow to have the emotional capacity to receive and respect others no matter the hardship at hand. I pledged to myself that I wouldn't get stuck on why things were happening. I could have easily gotten lost in a "why is this happening to me" mindset, but instead, I started looking for the lesson in what was showing up—in what was right in front of me. Investing time and energy in being angry and upset about the things that were happening around me was not productive. It wouldn't change anything either. So I chose to honor what was going on and decide how I would push through—no matter what came my way.

Affirmations for Being Unbothered

Read these out loud in a seated position.

I am rooted deeply in my truth.

I will not fall victim to the distraction of hatred.

I am in charge of myself and where my energy goes.

I am not bothered by things I cannot control.

I will control myself, my love, and my heart.

I am unbothered in the best way.

WHAT IT MEANS TO ME: Being unbothered isn't just something that I live by, it's something that I deeply believe brings me peace. Life has a funny way of testing us, and over the years I have had my fair share of being tested. However, deciding that certain things, people, and energies were not allowed into my space was a turning point. I became dedicated to self-control, love, and compassionate understanding. Hurt people have tried to hurt me. Broken people have tried to break me. I have not let either happen because my peace is protected by a divine source. I am whole in the face of destruction. I have a sound mind in the face of emotional unrest. I have learned to be unbothered so that my light isn't dimmed by darkness.

READER REFLECTION: Make a list of everything that is bothering you in your journal. Cross off the things that you cannot change at this very moment. Circle the things that you can change to-day. Start the things that are a work in progress. If you are on a quest to live an unbothered life, this practice can help you regain control of your emotions and focus on what you can change and what you cannot.

Being intentional is a choice that no one can take from you, even when they try their hardest. Facing the challenges of being on tour and seeing the news about my children's mother and a former band member seemingly everywhere I looked wasn't a walk in the park. I wasn't *not* upset—but I was more focused on my character and what responding versus reacting looked and felt like on a professional and personal level. It affected me in a profound way and in a multitude of ways. What I was becoming more aware of is the truth behind there always being two sides. On one side, everything coming to the surface was the necessary information that I needed to further my knowledge of self. It was the permission I needed to trust in myself more. I needed to be reminded of things that I saw that I overlooked. I needed my true self to step up and remind me of who I really was. Moving forward in grace was the display of good karmic energy I was putting out into the world, even during a really shitty time.

When the news came out about Dreux and April, everyone was looking to me to have this intense reaction. Rightfully so,

I could've easily fucked shit up. This was indeed an emotional thing to go through. Having millions of witnesses was pretty wild too. But reacting seldom gets us anywhere, especially when emotions are high. Being clear-minded so that I could be emotionally sound was my goal. And with much self-reflection and time to think, I had to take some responsibility for the things and behaviors I allowed to proceed. Mastering my emotions when handling this situation really matured me; it made me become a real man, not just the idea of one. I wouldn't have been able to respond in the way I did without having spent my twenties and beyond focusing on my spiritual development, prioritizing my physical wellness over being in the club all the time, honing my creative voice, and leaning into my role as a father. I imagine that if this had happened before I became more aware of the importance of staying grounded, things would have played out differently. Over the years, I had evolved and set out to be a man of dignity, respect, and good character—so even though I was dealing with such a public and humiliating thing, I was proud of myself for making the choice to not take the bait being offered. Hurt people hurt people. They'll often confuse love with dysfunction and chaos. So once I got clear on what was in front of me, it became easier not to take things personally.

THINGS ALWAYS
COME BACK AROUND:
YOU GET TO CHOOSE
WHAT GETS YOUR
ATTENTION AND ENERGY
AND WHAT DOESN'T.

I'm not saying I was perfect during this experience: I had mo-ments of frustration, being angry, and taking out pain on people around me, and overall not being my best self. I'm human. But what I'm saying is that I didn't let those feelings get the best of me, and I learned to master them through the tools I had learned over the years, whether it was a breath exercise when I was feeling particularly frustrated or going for a bike ride to channel the neg-ative energy in a productive way. It became more peaceful to not get distracted and, instead, carry on with love at the center. We have to remember, distractions do not allow us to think clearly and with open minds. It causes brain fog, a lack of openness and empathy, and inner chaos. Being clear and aligned with my high-est self was a radical choice. It was self-mastery. I don't know many men who would have the self-control to not react when going through a situation like this, let alone have to work alongside the person on a world tour. But I did, and how I handled this scandal was absolutely intentional.

| Energy Check: Being Unbothered

Why is it important to you to be unbothered?

Is being unbothered the best thing to do for every situation?

How important is your peace?

What makes being unbothered worth it?

How important is it to you to be in control of your emotions?

No one could pave the way for me. I had to be the prototype. I had to be the man and mentor that I wanted growing up. I had to choose that path. Everything I was walking through at the time pushed me to be a new person, a person I would be proud of. I would not allow certain things to throw me off track, even if it was happening maliciously. The clarity this brought to my life has reverberated into my business. It's taught me personal value and what it truly means to be committed to self. How we show up in the world is a reflection of so many things—our traumas, our joys, our failures, and our successes alike. Mastering my emotions was like a mirror to not just the outside world but also myself. Realizing the extension of power within myself changed a lot for me.

When I sat and thought about the type of impact I wanted to leave on the world, it became so much clearer that I have the power to set the tone for someone else's behavior. Even if they choose not to change, how I move through the world will at least give them something to think about. This intention can affect their story. Mastering my emotions taught me about leading by example for my kids. It continues to teach me valuable lessons on leadership. I've come to realize that when you lead by example, you create an idea of what's possible. People can look at you and say, *If he can do it, I can do it.* Leading by example has made it easy for others to see the different ways they can greet and learn from the adversity that shows up in their lives. When I learned where my roots were and what I was planted in, the harvest of my experiences was divine teachers and abundant creators. That alone commanded attention and created deeper integrity. If I allowed the negativity and poor actions of others to infiltrate my space, mastering my emotions would have been much harder. The entire process of learning how to be in tune with myself and my feelings, good and bad, pushed me forward and showed me how to get out of my own way. I discovered what it meant to truly focus on myself and be the best I could be despite what was in front of me.

While some may not understand this, everything I walked through with A'mei and Megaa's mom was a blessing. It brought me closer to my truth and reminded me of what I wanted and what I didn't. It made me more focused, committed, and clear. And not reacting out of anger, fear, or pain allowed space for true inner healing. Our healing is no one else's job but our own, but before we can truly dive into that truth, we have to make a choice. Hate, cheating, stealing, and intentional wrongdoing do not elevate love. Going back and forth and trying to prove a point is draining. I was committed to staying focused—not pulled down into a vortex of trauma and hurt. Something that I hold very close to my heart is remembering that everyone has learned love differently, be it in a clear and healthy way or in a confused and unhealthy way. There will be people in our lives who believe that love and pain are synonymous. When hurt is all you know in the face of love, it's easy to get confused. People, myself included, only have the emotional capacity to change when they are ready to.

| Energy Check: Master Your Emotions

What are some things that you can do to remain calm in an intense situation?

What are the benefits of doing deep breathing exercises?

How important is it to know when to express yourself?

When is it essential to give yourself space?

How can meditation support your emotional intelligence?

Over the years, I have grown to be so much more aware of myself, to the point that I can feel things coming before they arrive. So this situation wasn't a surprise to me. It was, however, a reminder to trust the feeling and things that present themselves, even if they're subtle. It's one thing to be aware of your emotions and intuition. It's another thing to do something about what you feel. And that attunement is where the boys get separated from the men. I'm not going to lie; this type of soul work is exhausting. It's so much easier to move through the world blindly than it is to move intentionally. It takes a lot of brainpower, energy, and awareness to really know yourself and enjoy your life. You have to energetically be sound. What I've come to know well on my journey is that true enjoyment is allowing things to just be, even the things we cannot control—even the things that may be hurting us. That is the centerpiece of mastering our emotions, cultivating inner peace. Being okay with whatever outcome, even if it's a trying one, offers up a sense of emotional ease. There is joy in surrendering and having trust in what we cannot change. This has been a great takeaway for me as a man and a father. The world may look at me as the king of being unbothered, but it's so much deeper than that. The importance of being unbothered is to exercise self-control and be aware of the people who purposely go out of their way to inflict pain, confusion, and reactionary energy on you.

Every day I am making a purposeful choice to not get swept up in the negative and toxic cycles of others. I try my best to not pay attention to things that don't serve me, and I don't take things personally. Projections are not my truth. I would much rather deal with issues head-on if it's serious enough, but more often than not I choose to protect my peace and keep moving. Every day I am committing to being the man that I needed growing up. I couldn't master my emotions if I wasn't also committed to not allowing certain things to have power over me. Being unbothered supported my peace of mind and showed me that sometimes how people treat us is less a reflection of us and more a reflection of them and their unresolved trauma. Not getting swept away in emotional currents puts me in a great position to be open to finding solutions and learning the beauty of acceptance.

Having this type of dedication and clarity around my choices and emotions is deeper than being unbothered. It's a lifestyle and commitment to deeply rooted freedom. I am liberated by my choice to not feed into the nonsense that others try to project on me. Being on tour with someone who was actively trying to disrupt my peace of mind was the test of a lifetime. It took discipline and willpower to not get distracted by dysfunctional behavior. Co-parenting with someone who didn't have the emotional capacity to be cordial and nonmanipulative, because of her own trauma, was beyond emotionally challenging. But I refused to let the toxicity and brokenness of someone else interrupt the intentional life I was dedicated to living. Mastering emotions is a true test of manifesting and adhering to inner harmony. If we let people and things not aligned with our highest self or good pull us down, we are destined to succumb to the pressure.

| BEING UNBOTHERED MEDITATION |

I am walking away from toxicity.

Be unbothered.

Sometimes we go far for people who deserve very little.

Be unbothered.

I am willing to find a new way or make one.

Be unbothered.

I am disrupting ignorance with clarity.

Be unbothered.

I will gather my thoughts, be honest with myself.

Be unbothered.

I know now all that matters is what is meant for me.

Be unbothered.

I know that some things are meant to be but not meant to last.

Be unbothered.

I stand firm in my truth like a rock undisturbed and unmoved.

Be unbothered.

Ignorance and rudeness crave attention and acknowledgment.

Be unbothered.

My peace of mind and the well-being of my children matter above all else. Over the years, the clearest takeaway I've uncovered is that checking in with ourselves, even under extreme circumstances, pressure, and stress, is pivotal to our growth. Being tested on tour and in my relationship with my ex made it clear that settling was not an option. I was not going to lose myself in hopes of finding answers that had nothing to do with me. Regardless of what was thrown my way, being emotionally reactionary would not have been conducive to my growth. I refused to engage in low-frequency behavior. Doing so would have gone against everything I had built for myself on a spiritual level—everything I was trying to show my children. Unhealthily reacting to what we cannot control does not create room for growth or change. Instead, it builds walls and barriers that are hard to dismantle.

What does create room for expansion and elevation is making the choice to stay focused and not take things so personally. Keeping a clear mind and perspective even when faced with obstacles allows for intentional problem-solving and acceptance when we don't have, or can't find, the answers we're looking for. Being unbothered and mastering my emotions has allowed me to sit in the discomfort and ask myself the hard questions: *What do I want? What matters the most to me? What will my children think?* Processing all of this has shown me that I deserve to pause and take a moment to recalibrate. Everything impactful takes time, even when we're working through conflict, discomfort, and negativity. I chose to stay grounded in peace because peace is bliss—and in the presence of emotional tranquility, we grow closer to the truth.

| Energy Check: Mastering Emotions

What has adversity taught you about yourself and how you respond to it?

Where do you need to slow down and pause in your life?

Who inspires you to be your best self?

What has love taught you about growing?

How are you learning to master your emotions?

LET LIFE WAKE YOU UP TO THE POSSIBILITIES BEFORE YOU.

5

Sex, Energy + Life Force

I started thinking more about sex and the energy tied to it in my twenties. I was searching for a new way to be present and to have a deeper connection to myself. Having women at my disposal got old, and to be honest, my energy wasn't aligned with my highest self. For three years, I embarked on a journey of celibacy, and it was by far one of the most trying and enlightening decisions I've made as a man. It was also hard as hell. And it's definitely not for everyone. Spiritually, I was ready to take on a new path and interconnectedness. I was in my midtwenties, a new homeowner, and had a live-in girlfriend. Talk about a challenge. I knew no one my age who would have chosen celibacy for themselves—but I'm built differently. When I put my mind to something, even if it means no sex, I stick to it. If it will elevate my mind, body, and soul, I am open to the possibilities and dedicated to showing up and doing the work. The decision to rid myself of sexual distraction shaped and afforded me the space and time to get clear about the man I wanted to be in the world. My goal with celibacy was to get closer to myself and truly understand the importance of what it meant to be close with a woman on an intimate and nonsexual level. Mind you, doing this with a live-in girlfriend made the task of no sex tempting to break. When I started learning that sex was linked to the energy that could lift up or drain, I started looking at my sexual relationships and partners differently. I was at a point in my life where whom I slept with mattered, for their sake and for mine. We were exchanging energy, good and bad. Soul ties are real. So being able to have self-control when it came to my sex life was empowering and commanded my full intention.

At that time, I was developing my spirituality and exploring the Jehovah's Witness religion. Me and my then girlfriend were embarking on that path together. I was devoted to strengthening my relationship with the Creator. When I was introduced to the organization of Jehovah's Witnesses, I was intrigued. That religious practice was completely different from anything that I've experienced. Growing up Baptist and enjoying birthday celebrations and holidays was what I was accustomed to. Jehovah's Witnesses were far from what I was familiar with. They don't celebrate holidays or birthdays. The music wasn't the same. And becoming a member required intense studying and knowledge before being able to be baptized. At the time, I was dedicated to learning how to have complete control over myself, my actions, and my mind. I was coming to the realization that I needed to release myself from outside judgment and regain inner clarity and perspective.

Being involved with the organization for those few years taught me the importance of discipline, inner power, and the ability to not allow sexual pleasure to consume me. This was one of the many religions I had explored over the years, and while it ended up not being for me, the lessons I learned really challenged me to get honest with myself about where I was investing my time and energy. What I've come to know through my experience is that if in fact sex is a sacred act, it should be an agreement rooted in respect and open communication. Prior to this realization, a lot of my sexual encounters were not in alignment with that. During this early spiritual experience, it became clear to me as a man that love and sex are not synonymous.

When I changed my mindset, I changed as a whole and for the better. For me, that looked like focusing on the ways I needed to be more in tune with my spirituality, mind, body, and soul. There was a point in time that having and entertaining different women was embedded in how I moved through the world. From being a musician and sex symbol to trying to break free from that stereotype took dedication. Most folks may think that's a crazy choice for someone in my position—but it wasn't crazy to me. Abstaining was a liberating experience. It was like I had started the voyage home to my true self, no detours. And yes, it was hard as hell. I love women and being with them, but my needs shifted. My mind was clearer. Everything started to make more sense. Being mindful about the energy I was sharing with people changed the game for me. As a man, it was important for me to be cognizant of where not only my sexual energy was going, but also my emotional and spiritual energy.

LIFE FORCE MEDITATION

I am reinvigorated.

I make.

I hold.

I obtain.

I am.

I conduct.

I am a force.

I lead.

I create.

I am.

I expand.

I am omnipresent.

I shift.

I grow.

I am.

I have the power over myself.

I believe.

I trust.

I authentically exist.

I am.

I draw energy from the earth.

I uplift.

I recharge.

I transform.

I am a reflection of the Universe.

Abstaining from sex woke me up spiritually. It allowed me to tap into a newfound discipline and self-awareness, especially when it pertained to pleasure. I think it's easy to get joy and pleasure confused. What I've learned is that there's a difference between the two. Pleasure is fleeting and momentary. Joy, on the other hand, is something that offers stability within ourselves. I was noticing that a lot of men, including myself, weren't attuned to being fully present with women, romantically or platonically. We were also lacking the emotional capacity to be fully present with ourselves. Intense emotions that come with lust and sex can be distracting to our detriment.

Taking a step back to see things more clearly in my sexual relationships made room for me to pay closer attention to my platonic and familial relationships as well. Every step of this process opened me up to new ways of thinking and processing my relationships. I became more open to learning thoughtfulness, acceptance, and understanding of women on a more aligned level. All of this is vital because so often there is a disconnect between the two. Investing my energy intentionally and where it counts the most has allowed me to become more clear about using it wisely in all facets of my life.

| Energy Check: Sex, Energy + Life Force

What is the importance of drinking alkaline water?

How can you improve your energy by the foods you ingest?

What kind of boundaries are you setting for yourself to conserve your energy?

What methods can you use to recharge your energy?

Is it beneficial to you to share your sacred energy with everyone?

Stepping back into the real world, where sex is seemingly not a big deal, I was tempted left and right. And if I'm being honest, I had my share of backtracking and having a wild moment or two.

I wasn't sure what I wanted, to be in a relationship or to date. But I did know that I was ready to not be celibate. I had spent so much time in celibacy that I said "fuck it": I learned what I needed. It was in that moment that really showed me how important my celibacy journey was. I went from nothing to everything, and it shook me up. I felt all over the place and needed to recenter. After breaking away from the no sex life, shit came at me fast. And it was then that I truly realized that connecting mentally with women versus only sexually was what I longed for. In or out of a relationship. Having my fuck-it moment made me realize that I needed and wanted more than a physical connection. That was where my true desire lived. Things became more apparent, and I had to start practicing the intention that I learned during my celibacy season.

I learned that a woman must appeal to me more than just by how she looks. Mentally, I knew I needed and wanted to be stimulated, mind, body, and soul. Being physically attracted to a woman is great, but is there an emotional connection for us to talk, have fun together, go places without it just being about intimacy? Men aren't taught how to move through the world in this way often enough. We are encouraged and celebrated to get the girl, fuck her, and keep it moving. That's what makes us a man, that's what makes us *the* man. The takeaway from celibacy taught me that that shit wasn't where it was at and that lifestyle gets old quick. I mean, when I got back in the having-sex game, it was clear that I had outgrown that behavior even when I decided to push back and revert to old ways. Don't get me wrong, the sex was good, but the lack of connection wasn't often worth the temporary pleasure.

I believe that we should have, enjoy, and experience sexual pleasure, but there comes the point in our lives where there is more to it than that. Without my journey through celibacy, I wouldn't have had the emotional maturity to decipher the two. The experiences of knowing what it felt like to intentionally choose not to have sex with women changed how I looked at relationships and intimately connecting on a deeper mental level. Seeing that there were other ways that I could connect with women was pivotal for me and my growth as a man.

| Energy Check: Journal Prompts

Are you willing to give up things in order to get what you want? If so, what are they?

Are you happy where you are today?

Where do you want to grow and change in your life?

How do you practice self-love?

What are you trying to attract in your life?

Experiencing both sides of the path really showed me what kind of person I wanted to be. Even though I'm not practicing celibacy anymore or in a committed relationship, I carry the lessons from that point in my life close. I know myself well enough now to check in with my energy before sharing it with someone else. I've noticed that if I'm just linking up with someone physically, energetically I'm not really feeling like myself. I'm off my path, so to speak. And if anything, I'm likely going to be more drained of my energy after our encounter. There have been many hard lessons learned from having sex when I shouldn't have. Sharing our sexual energy with people should be an intentional act, even if it is just pleasure driven. We all have to learn this eventually—with age and time comes wisdom and clarity.

As we find ourselves on the path of sex, energy, and its connection to our life force, I want men to realize how powerful our sexual energy is. Being intentional is key to growth and a deeper understanding of ourselves and others. The people we connect with become an extension of us. Taking responsibility for our sexual energy and wellness is crucial. Fucking isn't the only way to prove you're "man enough." I'm not here to judge anybody, but I am here to give my fellow man something to think about and consider. While I believe that everyone should have the space and opportunity to freely express themselves, it's definitely important to manage our energy mindfully. I wouldn't know this to be true if I didn't have my own wake-up calls, failures, shortcomings, and missteps along the way. I've experienced both sides of the spectrum. If I hadn't, I wouldn't be able to see why being measured and mindful in all that I do, especially when it comes to sex, is a must.

Celibacy as a choice for men isn't discussed regularly. It's no secret that we are raised and taught to find our value in sex, to flex our masculinity, to have as many women on our roster as possible. I was tired of that shallow way of thinking. It's easy to think with your dick; it's much more challenging to be mindful about whom you share sexual energy with. The reason we don't have some of the things we want in life is that we refuse to sacrifice and get uncomfortable.

I've been there and have had to learn the hard way many times. Being celibate for three years, I learned deep self-control and became more aware of my energetic footprint. I wasn't perfect. The urge to have sex wasn't nonexistent: it was very much alive and well. But just because the urge was there didn't mean I was going to act on it. Where my energy was going and flowing started to mean more and more to me each passing day. Spiritually I evolved into a person willing to give things up to transform into my highest self. We have to let go in order to gain. We can't expect true change if we're stuck on staying the same and not challenging ourselves, our thoughts, and our beliefs.

I connected with a deep sense of growth and transformation during this chosen path. Being willing to take on the challenge to abstain was a true act of self-love for me. I wasn't taught this growing up, and a lot of folks would have looked at me sideways if they knew I was sacrificing sex for inner peace and clarity. That point in my life showed me how to have *inner* pleasure and joy. I was elevating and becoming better for myself, and with that, I was also giving myself permission to change on a more intentional level. Everything I thought I knew shifted. I was emotionally expanding in a way I hadn't before. I was getting to know my true self and also gaining the knowledge around being okay with being alone. I was slowly learning how to trust myself and find inner strength through discernment.

As a society, there is a stigma around choosing not to have sex for whatever reason. I learned that many men have chosen to abstain in an effort to reclaim their energy and exercise discipline to become a more enlightened version of themselves. Ultimately, we are the only ones who can decide to accept that change is necessary to our well-being. That change for most won't be giving up sex, but it was for me.

The power to live in the fullness of life is a divine choice and that choice looks different for each of us. Now, I'm not saying to give up sex and walk into a light of celibacy, but I am saying that when you know what's draining you, you can start taking the steps to repair what needs to be repaired. I'm the type of person who enjoys challenges and taking on things that are deemed "hard to do." And while this no-sex choice wasn't easy by any means, it offered me clarity, a deeper connection to myself and romantic interests, and it allowed me to turn away from the immediate satisfaction of life and get introspective about the long-term goals I had. I was open to learning how to be one with myself, and I've found that so many other men have taken on the task of doing the same. Women are amazing and I enjoy having sex—but I was steadfast in the decision to find belonging and true joy within myself. I was committed to discovering a connection with the opposite sex on a more authentic level.

My greatest takeaway while abstaining was that I am in control of how I show up in the world. Sex is a magical act; so often, we are not with the right partners and we are exchanging emotional and sexual energy that is toxic. Being able to get clear about this taught me that I can create the world I want inside myself. And it was an open invitation to figure out how to create healthy sexual bonds with women that weren't rooted in a shallow way of thinking. In turn, that translated to the energy I attracted outside myself. Another key takeaway is that there is no task too great for me to handle. Being a man, to me, means being able to discern, be disciplined, and stay committed to what's important. If I could go without sex, I could master anything. I was willing to give up something I enjoyed to get what I wanted: *a more aligned self-loving, a more meaningful life.* I was open to changing, growing, and outgrowing to connect with a deeper knowledge of self-awareness and happiness in my life. Everything isn't supposed to be easy, and embarking on the road of celibacy showed me that first hand, in the very best way.

Affirmations for Sex, Energy + Life Force

Read these out loud in a seated position.

My energy is sacred.

I will invest my time wisely.

My love is sacred.

I will be mindful of the company I keep.

My life force is sacred.

I will take care when sharing my time and energy with others.

I am deserving of love.

WHAT IT MEANS TO ME: Where my energy goes is important. My time and love are sacred. There was a time when I wasn't mindful of where my energy was going and flowing. The more I've matured, it's become very clear that where I spend my time, invest my love, and share my energy matters. This affirmation serves as a reminder to stay clear about the intentions I've set over the years when it comes to preserving the most sacred parts of myself and life.

READER REFLECTION: What is sacred to you in your life? How can you protect your time and energy more effectively? Where are you wasting your time and energy?

A SOURCE OF MY
POWER IS THE ABILITY
TO LET THINGS GO AND
ENJOY THE MOMENTS
WHILE THEY LAST.

LIFE WILL TEACH US HOW
TO BE IN TUNE WITH
OURSELVES.

| CLARITY MEDITATION |

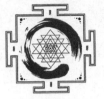

I am calling in clarity for emotional expansion.

I am calling in clarity to create the necessary boundaries in my life to be at ease.

I am calling in clarity for a more open heart and mind.

I understand that a lack of clarity can cause confusion, stress, and communication roadblocks.

I understand that in order to live and lead the life I want, clarity must be a welcomed friend.

When clarity emerges in my life, it allows me to free up energy that would otherwise be a hindrance.

A moment of clarity feels like time is standing still.

Clarity increases my trust and transparency.

Clarity is knowing exactly what I want.

To see the path is to be the path.

Clarity identifies what matters and eliminates my distractions.

Clarity shows my mind and heart confirmation.

I am calling in abundant clarity.

Be mindful. Be thoughtful. Have courage.

6

Start Where You Are

I create my own path and walk it in blissfully.

I create.

I have the courage to try new things and excel in them.

I create.

Today I will make progress toward my goals.

I create.

Negative thoughts only have power if I let them.

I create.

I will use what I have and do whatever I can.

I create.

I will be expansive and not limit myself.

I create.

I will not let expectations or the opinion of others distract my focus.

I create.

I will be available to serve my purpose.

I create.

I remember the LA night scene—the early 2000s—when it was important to be seen in the flesh. There was Playhouse, Supper Club, and Greystone Manor; they were the hottest spots in the city at the time. In my late twenties, life was a party. LA is a special place with so many cultures and people to connect with. I was living my life to the fullest.

Before having my son, Megaa, my life was all about being an entertainer and being seen. The club was a middle ground where my celebrity and normalcy could meet. I was young, childfree, and enjoying the freedom of being able to do what I wanted when I wanted. Being on the scene was exciting. I lived in Hollywood at the time—1600 Vine Street—a very vibrant and diverse place to be. Living in the heart of Hollywood was wild. The partying, the noise, the being out and about—I got tired of it. It became stale. The clubs were filled with the same people, the same music, and it started to feel like there was nothing for me there. There was a constant rotation of the same crowd linking up and out-of-towners looking for a good time. I started asking myself, *What am I doing here?* I was hanging out with the DJs at the clubs every weekend getting my records played but feeling more uninspired to be there every time. There was a pulling need to always be out and in the mix because I spent my young adult life being one of the most famous lead singers in a mainstream group. So I thought it was a part of my job and duty as a performer to not only show up onstage but off the stage as well.

Back in the 2000s, it was the norm to be out socializing with actors, producers, and other celebrities. We all wanted to be seen in some capacity. There was a thrill to it all—the VIP sections, the women, the drinking, the glitz and glamour that few get to experience in this lifetime. Over time, I had developed this level of mystique as an artist to be in connection with the outside world, to know what's going on, but also to be in my own lane. When I was hanging out, I was hanging out big time. Sometimes I would get booked to do walk-throughs at the clubs, which felt like my own personal party. I was treated like a king, everyone knew my name, and everyone wanted O in the building. And even though I slowly started to feel this pull to step away from that life, at times I felt it was necessary to be out because you never know who you might cross paths with. There was always someone new to meet and connect with. In those days, if you weren't out and partying and showing off, you weren't really a star. I didn't want to miss anything, and a part of me didn't want to be forgotten.

Going out all the time took a toll on my body. I wasn't a heavy drinker, but taking a little drink here and there each time started to add up. Alcohol was a big part of the culture. If you were out, you were drinking because everyone was. That was the thing to do. Even though I wasn't a super-heavy drinker, my body showed me that you don't have to be to witness and experience the impact that alcohol can have on a person internally and externally. A combination of no rest and no water will make anyone look dehydrated and bloated. My body was not what it used to be, and it showed. I looked at myself in the mirror and said, *Hold up, this isn't sexy O. This isn't the person I want to see looking back at me.* That was my turning point, seeing how I lost touch with my physical wellness and fitness chasing a lifestyle and a scene that I didn't really want in the first place. Starting fresh felt like the best option. I was ready to transform myself. I was ready to let go of the party life, drinking, and not taking good care of myself.

After having my son, Megaa, at thirty, I was inspired to embark on the journey of returning back to myself—but as an even better version. I believe in leading by example and teaching our children, who are always watching how to be—by actions, not just by words. A mutual friend introduced me to Scott Parker, aka Scotty P, who is a master trainer and life experience coach. He's changed my life and has played a major role in showing me many things about myself and others. Not long after we met, Scott introduced me to the bike trail. I didn't envision biking becoming a forever hobby for me, but it has. The first ride we did was about eight miles. At the time, that was pretty impressive because I was reestablishing my childhood joy of riding a bike and transforming it into adult freedom of productivity.

I became completely engulfed with bike riding, being outside in nature, and being physically active again. I was in love and ready to take on this new and beautiful challenge. After eight miles we did twelve, after twelve we did twenty, and after twenty we did twenty-eight. I was hooked. I felt like I could ride for days on end. We eventually worked our way up to forty miles, and I had discovered newfound freedom.

This was the life I wanted, needed, and had been missing. My longest ride is fifty-one miles. Riding clears my mind. I'm able to process unanswered questions and be in the moment. Biking offered me a much-needed reset to focus on my spiritual, physical, and mental health. I didn't know what I was getting into when I hopped on the bike as an adult. But I quickly realized that the recommitment to myself was what I'd been longing for. I'm able to encourage myself when I ride. I'm able to be inspired and creative. That was something I was missing. The night scene wasn't giving me that. The drinking wasn't offering me any type of emotional clarity. Reconnecting with my body was a gift. Some of the best ideas come to me while I'm riding. I am my most creative and free self while on the bike. I learn something from everything around me, the weather, the terrain, and the breathtaking beauty of nature.

Changing my life in this way showed me that I could do anything and everything that I committed myself to. Be it not drinking or dedicating myself to myself. To think that if I wouldn't have reevaluated myself that day in the mirror, I may have never been brave or curious enough to try an old thing like bicycling in a new way. It's easier to stay the same than it is to make active and intentional changes that will set us up for longevity in the long run. On our journeys through change, we have to be self-aware enough to move away from what's keeping us stuck and move toward what's going to challenge us.

Partying and drinking were keeping me stuck in a low vibrational way of living. I believe in having fun, but I also believe in finding ways to balance fun with mental and physical fitness. Life is about trying new things and not getting stuck in old bad habits that do not serve or uplift us. It's a true joy to be able to start where you are even when it's challenging the hell out of us. When we're open to new beginnings, that means we're also open to growth. When we're open to a challenge, that means we're open to the lessons and takeaways of failing or succeeding. Each is an opportunity to raise your vibration, cultivate self-belief, and trust in your ability as great as you say you are.

| Energy Check: Start Where You Are

Are you open to learning new things?

What are your goals?

How will you handle adversity?

What problem will you solve?

How important is it to strategize?

EACH STEP IN MY
JOURNEY HAS SHAPED
MY OVERALL PURPOSE
AND PRIORITIES IN LIFE.
CHANGE IS BEAUTIFUL,
AND IT PREPARES
US FOR A FRUITFUL
FUTURE.

Meeting Scott Parker was a turning point in my transformation at age thirty. I told him that I wanted to transform my body and get back to a healthier state. He was ready to help me take on the challenge and get right. This was a deeply personal choice on many levels, not just for vanity but for my overall health and well-being. I prided myself in looking a certain way as an entertainer, but I also knew it was in my interest to stop drinking so that I could feel my best on a holistic level. I had fallen off a bit, but I was ready to get back to my best and healthiest self. I was up for the challenge and ready to do the work to get back in shape.

Taking that first step was rejuvenating. I had been at my best before, and I was dedicated to getting back there. Starting deserves to be celebrated. It's no small feat to do things that are hard or feel out of reach. The choice to change came into my life in divine time. I believe that every thought and pull on the heart to change happens in perfect timing. Not long after I made this decision to shift into a better physical version of myself, I found out I would become a father for the first time. That was a pivotal moment in my life, business, and career. I was so excited to step into fatherhood. I was ready and couldn't wait to be a dad. Everything felt anew in an instant. I had rediscovered what it meant to be fully present—not only for myself but for someone else, my child.

Becoming a father was a whole new start in itself. I had no idea how to raise a kid, but I was absolutely going to do my best in that sacred role. As unfamiliar as I was with parenthood, I was absolutely ready to take on the job. I knew that I needed to prepare myself to be responsible for a whole human being. I did not take that responsibility lightly. I knew for a fact that I wanted to be, and would be, the man that my son would look to with pride as I raised him. When I look back, it's interesting to see that this major life change was coming on the heels of making the decision to take better care of myself. This wasn't a coincidence; it was aligned with my highest good on so many levels. And I truly believe that my entire experience—from dedicating myself to my wellness to becoming a father—was linked in the best way for me to become my best self.

I also began to pay closer attention to my value, productivity, and effort. As I was changing and evolving into this new version of myself, physically and emotionally, I found myself having more inner dialogue conversations. I would start to question who was around me, where I needed to shift, and who I needed to let go of. I was looking at all of these little tedious things and asking myself, *Does this person value me? If I wasn't who I was, would this person support me?* I was taking a real close look at everything in my life. Once I took that first bike ride and rode those eight miles, clarity started flooding in. It was at that moment, with this new experience, that I could make a mindful choice to start over. To begin again and redirect my life toward deeper alignment. I had become committed to pushing myself to the limit to be my best, on the bike and off the bike, in fatherhood and in my individuality as a man. Things were changing in the best way for me, and

I'm not sure this new awakening would have presented itself in this way if I hadn't started biking with Scott.

A whole new world was waiting for me. Changing started to be second nature—it felt good to choose something different for myself. I started looking at the ending of my old life, relationships, and ways as just the beginning of something greater and more magnificent. We have to learn and trust to be okay with those new beginnings and not quite knowing where to go. There are lessons in exploring new ways of finding yourself and trusting the path that you're on, today, at this moment. I believe that everyone needs motivation. We all need a reason to really tap into a stride that is unstoppable. My son gave me the motivation to go beyond the limits I had put on myself. So as I continued to grow into my best self for this greater purpose, I became invigorated by knowing that I was leading by example. I wasn't willing to wait for anybody to give me permission to change. It had to start with me and my determination to be who I said I wanted to be. My life wasn't just about me anymore. I was proudly paving a new way.

Between biking and fatherhood, my evolution was on the horizon. I learned that changing has to be an intentional choice and part of the human process to learn what's working and what is not. It's necessary in life to face ourselves and evolve into our best. We cannot solely commit to doing something different. We have to put action behind that commitment. Looking at myself in the mirror all those years ago, and not liking what I saw, was my starting point. Actively committing to take care of myself showed me how strong I really am. And even when I didn't think that biking was going to be a revolutionary change for me, I tried it and realized that it's just what I needed to deepen the commitment I had made to myself.

My son coming into my life deepened my willingness to learn and be better too. There have been so many layers to starting over and taking on the task of doing something new even without the expertise. The point of life is to learn and be open to the lessons that present themselves. Each step in my journey has shaped my overall purpose and priorities in life. Change is beautiful, and it prepares us for a fruitful future. It allows us to take on things we may have never thought we had the power to do. I have a new perspective and outlook. I feel that this is what life is about: my music, changing in my body and overall wellness, and being a father.

When I think about all the information streams of life and experience, it's showing me something new. It's all reminding me that I am forever growing and expanding for the greater good— and for that I am grateful. No one can prepare us for the lives we're destined to live. We have to prepare ourselves. It takes practice to become who we are destined to be. There will be moments when we don't know how to get started, and I think the most important thing we can do in those moments is to start anyway. We were built to begin again if we need to, to start fresh, or even to start something new for the first time. There is a lot of beauty in choosing to change, grow, and dive into a life that is worth living.

IF YOU DON'T
UNDERSTAND YOUR
VALUE, YOU CAN'T
REALLY HAVE A FULL
UNDERSTANDING AND
EXPERIENCE OF LIFE.

| Energy Check: Journal Prompts

Where do you need more discipline in your life?

What are your wellness goals?

Who inspires you to be a better version of yourself?

Forgiveness Mantra

I forgive myself for causing pain and suffering to myself and others.
I release.

I forgive myself for making mistakes.
I release.

I am building a future based on compassion and kindness.
I release.

I forgive myself for not speaking up when necessary.
I release.

I forgive myself for not understanding.
I release.

I forgive others for lack of knowledge.
I release.

I release self-resentment, hurt, and anger from my soul.
I transform.

PART 3 |

MENTAL

Infinite Possibilities + The Power of Choice

One of the most important things to realize about relationships is that we all have different paths in life. A good example is the transition from high school to college. Most of the time, this is where you part ways with your high school friends and take on a new identity as an individual. As we all know so well, everything changes. And in that change, growth starts to take place yet again. If we are to really do this life right, we must remember that growing and expanding is necessary to live a life of inner clarity and understanding. Heading toward a new path is infinitely on the horizon, waiting for us to journey forward and step into our power.

As I've embarked on my path of healing, growth, and learning, I've realized that wishing others well, even when our pathways are different, improves a sense of connectedness. I believe that there can be closeness in parting ways and growing in different directions. I believe this allows room for openness, clarity, and understanding. This belief counteracts one of the worst aspects of suffering and feeling alone in the growth and expansion that we all face in life. Both professionally and personally, learning that not everyone will grow with me was essential to me becoming more patient and open with my process. It also made room for me to understand and trust the power in letting go. One moment comes to mind, vividly, even years later. It woke me up pretty fast to just how different everyone's path, purpose, and life walk is.

The first bodyguard I had was a protector in my life. We met while I was just getting started in B2K, and he kept me safe on tour. We moved as a unit. My safety was his responsibility and priority. When we were on the road, I always felt safe, but when off-season came around, I was thrust into, what seemed like, fending for myself. When touring was up, he would go back home and be with his family and take care of his own life. I had gotten used to being on the road with him, and we became family. Touring and being away from loved ones can feel isolating at times. So having someone around who not only protected me but also understood me was major. When it was time for B2K to split and go our separate ways, none of the team worked for us anymore, except the security. He came with me into my solo career and stayed with me for a while. Then he started a family, moved to Atlanta, and we haven't worked together since then. That feels strange, but at the same time, it's a part of this business.

You learn to grow and go with the flow. Life can feel fast-paced and things can shift quickly, and this is something that I had to learn really early on. There have been a lot of changes in my career. People have come and gone—and I have learned over the years an entirely new process on how to respect people and honor the changes that show up in my life. Parting ways isn't always a tumultuous thing. Having people grow and move in different directions doesn't always mean something bad happened. There are instances where moving on is a must and in the best interest of everyone involved. Sometimes we are only meant to be in one another's lives for a short amount of time, and there is beauty in that. There will always be people who come into your life for a season versus a lifetime.

Thinking back to my time with B2K, I realize that that really intense time made me see things and people differently. There were so many foul things being said about me at an age when I didn't have the words or emotional maturity to speak up for myself. I was only seventeen years old. There were so many things that I wanted to say and didn't. Moving through the world feeling like I had to defend myself and my lane left me feeling like I was not sure how to react. I had to often ask myself, *How do you feel about this?* to get the clarity I was trying to find. During that time, after the B2K split, I saw this other lane that I could take versus reacting to the negativity around me. That lane led me to personal forgiveness. Self-forgiveness for not doing what I didn't know how to do open up an entirely new opportunity to connect to myself and become a better and more clear-minded person. I realized that other people's projections onto me were not mine to carry or worry about. They weren't disadvantages to me. And when I realized that I didn't have to take on and carry around other people's baggage and shit, I found inner peace.

I was a young man when I had this realization, and I've carried it with me ever since. Looking at how people handle things showed me that everyone doesn't have the capacity to be a positive force in this life. Dysfunction comes from somewhere, and not participating in the dysfunction of others changed the game. Not only did it show me the power of growth, forgiveness, and letting go, it's also been a great teacher on what not to do. Everyone doesn't have the capacity to do or be better even when we want them to. Remembering that that comes from somewhere, likely an unhealed part of themselves, makes it easier for me to not take things personally but instead work on understanding myself better. Growth lives in that space and time.

When I examined everything in front of me, I realized that even when I wanted to respond in a way that wouldn't support my highest self, choosing not to made me understand how controlling myself really mattered. Going off and letting my anger speak for me wasn't going to help me or resolve things. That can be hard as hell not to do when your name and reputation are on the line, but again—growth. Staying close to my truth and how I was the best thing I could've done for myself. Looking back, I was preparing for my spiritual path. I hadn't discovered meditation and breathwork yet, but I was well on my way.

| Energy Check: Forgiveness

How does forgiveness affect our overall health and mental well-being?

Why should you forgive someone who has caused you harm?

Why is forgiveness important?

Are you willing to let go and deal with your true feelings?

What is the power of forgiveness?

Fast-forward to after the breakup of B2K: I was able to really step into my growth when I sat down to talk to JBoog for the first time since parting ways with the group. My life had taken on an entirely new shape. I was successful, my solo career was amazing, and I had grown as a man. There had been so much shit said about me over the years, so when Boog asked to sit down and talk, I was interested in hearing what he had to say. I also felt that it would be beneficial for me to move on by having a sense of closure that this conversation could offer. This opportunity was me making an important and intentional choice to let go and attempt to move forward.

What a lot of people don't know, because we don't talk about it, is that we were being manipulated by an elder we had once trusted. A lot of the foul shit that was happening was taking place because of him pitting us against one another. It was disgusting and terrible to see such drama unfold at the hand of someone we all once trusted. Everyone knew this at the time, and it was no surprise. When someone's goal is to divide, conquer, and destroy, there's no stopping them. For a long time, this person was successful in doing just that. I believe that in time the dark comes to the light, and there's no need to be violent or act out of character, even when you may want to—because karma always has the last say.

Deciding to sit down with JBoog, I had hoped, would pave the way to not rekindling old feuds but fostering mutual respect and understanding for each other. It had been some years, the dust had settled, and I figured the time was now or never, especially since going on tour was on the table. I came to the conversation owning the fact that I knew who I was, regardless of what had been said about me. All I could do was show up as my best self with my truth in hand—nothing else mattered at the end of the day. I won't go into the details of our conversation, since it is between the two of us, but I will say it gave me clarity about a lot of things. Our conversation gave me closure and helped me unlock the truth about everything that was going on.

I think a lot about what helped me choose to get in the car that day to meet with JBoog, and a lot of it was rooted in my perspective that the best weapon we can have in any adverse or complicated situation is *how* we respond to things. This takes emotional intelligence and openness to see things from a different perspective. Something that helped me was when I stopped worrying about how things would work or end up—and instead started to focus on myself, my actions, and my emotions. Being in tune and aligned with ourselves is how we can start sowing the seeds of growth and emotional expansion.

Reflecting on my conversation with JBoog and how everything happened with B2K, I realize that not holding grudges is something that liberated me. For so long, I was pissed. They did me dirty and that shit was not okay with me. But at the end of the day, the anger I was holding toward them was keeping me from growing into my highest self. Not letting go was keeping me caught up in a whirlwind of dysfunction. As I grew into the man I wanted to be, I had to look at my past relationships, both personal and professional. I had to choose to free up my energy and release myself from those toxic cycles.

Unhealthy emotional entanglements will keep you trapped and stunted—and that is no way to live. If we don't make room in our lives for letting go, we end up draining our life force. It is imperative that we let go of things that are no longer serving us or our growth. Not holding grudges has helped me keep my focus sharp. It's allowed me to get closer to my self-awareness and continue on the path of liberating myself. I've been given the opportunity to imprint, impress, and have an impact on those who are watching from the sidelines. The B2K fallout was a shit show, the world saw us rise and fall, but I think what's been really eye-opening for me has been staying close to my truth, character, and integrity.

My journey to being unbothered started when I chose to not give a fuck about the things I couldn't change. That alone freed up my energy and allowed me more space to grow and become better all around. Moving through hurdles and then choosing to move on is powerful. Holding on to things we can't change manifests itself in our bodies. Carrying things that are not conducive to our well-being and emotional freedom will weigh us down and keep us distracted. So when I talk about being unbothered, what I'm really saying is give yourself permission to be liberated.

Affirmations for Growth

Read these out loud in a seated position.

I am always growing.

If I pay attention to my feelings, I can create a life that is meaningful and fruitful.

My growth will require letting go.

I will release what no longer serves me so that I can live in abundance and alignment.

WHAT IT MEANS TO ME: We are always growing, and I know that may feel uncomfortable. However, we can become our best selves in the throes of our growing pain. I believe that growing through hardship is a great teacher and is an opportunity to relinquish control. We will not grow forward if we are committed to staying the same and stuck in old bad habits. Living our best life requires active and intentional growth, even when things are hard.

READER REFLECTION: Where do you see yourself in five years? What would you like to have? Where would you like to be? Create a mini vision board in your journal and see what comes up. Think as big as you can. Then make notes about how you plan to get what you're longing for. You have to work for the growth and life you want; nothing is handed to you. Manifestation without work and making changes is just wishful thinking.

Knowing my role in life is what keeps me from walking around aimlessly. The roles of creator, protector, and parent keep me grounded. That's been a great takeaway lesson for me in manhood. When I look back, I can see that so many people have no idea what their purpose is and because of that, growth feels out of reach. What I want more of us to understand is that we get to choose how we want to live and move through the world. A small example here would be me sitting down to talk to Boog after years of misunderstanding and harsh words. I could have decided that doing something like that would be a waste of time and energy. I could have continued to have the attitude of "fuck them n———s" and not cared at all if we made amends. JBoog could have easily done the same. But instead, we decided that having a conversation would be best for moving forward. That was an intentional choice and gave us space to clear the air as much as we could. Unfortunately, at that time, nothing became of that conversation because it simply wasn't time. It wasn't until almost a decade later when we spoke again that we would go on to perform together for the Millennium Tour with a little more clarity and a little less hesitation.

That influenced my purpose and my work. And it allowed me a chance to reflect, grow, and live in alignment with how I had grown to be. When we realize who we are as individuals, we can take note of the role that we play in our own lives and the lives of others. We are interconnected and linked to one another's stories. As we choose to grow forward with this at the center of our lives, we can start to realize and see just how we will be remembered in this life. Everything we do is paving the way for the legacy we will leave behind.

Growing and changing have taught me so much about who I am and who I want to be. There have been many full-circle moments in my life that have served as reminders to keep evolving. Over the years, my character and integrity have been questioned, but I continue to remember who I am through it all. Integrity has helped me authentically engage with the value of my being. It's allowed me to conjure up and put together an aura that represents positivity. Not because things are always positive and glorious in my life but because I choose to live in the promising possibility that our inner light has to offer. As humans, we can get caught up in our darkness, in what is happening to us. But what I've taken away from that is there's power in choosing to not forget who you are even when others do. I believe that my integrity speaks to the class of a man, father, and business owner I am. No one can create a story about me that can overshadow my truth and integrity as a man—even when they try. And that, to me, is growth. That to me speaks volumes to how far I have come in this life. There is something extraordinary about being so whole that no matter what, no one can dismantle what you've built.

I've been shown so much on my path of staying committed to myself and my journey. I've discovered what it means to stand firm in my soundness of mind and spirit. That, to me, is growing on a divine level. Seeking completeness has defined and solidified how I need to grow as a man, and it's also shown me how to let go of what no longer serves me or leaves me feeling incomplete or on shaky ground. Soundness, completeness, and wholeness shape me as an artist, a father, a son, and so much more. Growing and evolving requires sacrificing. It's allowed me to create balance in my work life and personal life. From each situation of change that I've faced, the key takeaway is that people and paths will change—even if you feel like you're on the same path for ten years, your path can change. And if you are on the right track, growth and shedding will happen, because in reality, staying the same rarely happens.

There is always the possibility to do better, be better, and let go of what no longer serves us. Letting go of who we once were to step into who we truly are is a part of life. Growth is always a part of true evolution. Stay on the right side of your decisions and close to *your* truth. It is necessary, no matter what you face, to be able to stand up for yourself and recognize who you are and who you will be. The entire process of growth will encourage us to take a closer look at what kind of legacy and life we want to leave behind. Getting sidetracked will stunt your growth. There will always be outside forces trying to distract you from standing in your power; choosing to leave them outside your space will help you in the long run. I believe in accepting that growth can show us how we need to become better—even in discomfort. The more we realize that we need growth and expansion in our lives, the closer we will get to our truth and highest self.

REMEMBER TO STAY CLOSE TO YOUR CHARACTER. DOING SO IS NOT ONLY HOW YOU'RE SEEN BUT ALSO HOW YOU ARE FELT. BEING HONORABLE AND HONEST IN YOUR WORK AND YOUR RELATIONSHIPS IS ESSENTIAL TO LIVING A MEANINGFUL LIFE.

| Energy Check: Journal Prompts

Write a letter to your Growth and give gratitude for how far you've come. This may feel challenging, especially if you feel like you're not where you want to be. However, this exercise will help you remember that nothing happens overnight, and being a work in progress is also a part of the journey.

Where do you want to grow in your life?

Where have you grown? What has that growth, the highs and lows, taught you about standing in your truth and power?

8

Growth

In early 2021, I was at an iconic studio, called the Record Plant, recording songs for a new project. The room I was working in is renowned for being used by artists of a certain caliber. Chris Brown and I actually recorded his "Post to Be" verse there. It was good to be back in the room that birthed the biggest record that I have to date. "Post to Be" is a four-time multi-platinum song. This room and place are very special. In the room next door, during my reunion visit, Ron and Ernie Isley were there working on a new album. I hadn't seen or spoken to Ron Isley in years. The last time I saw him was when I recorded the "Girlfriend" video with B2K in 2002. Ron was one of B2K's biggest supporters all those years ago, and it felt serendipitous that we were in the same recording studio almost twenty years later. I sat in that recording booth thinking about divine timing and the power of being infinitely aligned with what is meant for me. A lot of the time, I feel like we as people can get caught up in how things should be and how we want them to be. But everything isn't congruent with our plans. Over time, my career and life experiences have taught me that things will shift and change. And I cherish knowing that there is where beauty is.

When Ron Isley saw me, it was all love. We chopped it up, and he played me his new album. With him being a living legend, I've always admired and valued what he brings to the art of music and performing. At that time, watching him at almost eighty years old still have the magic touch and unwavering talent showed me that the career I wish to have as I age and change is possible. Ron was looking fly and fresh. He was still in the studio making hits. Witnessing that left a lasting impression on me. It shifted my perspective and gave me hope that I can continue to transform through my art regardless of my age.

Watching Ron showed me that I don't have to get old with music. I can thrive and stay invigorated by my craft and by the sounds around me. As Ron was leaving the studio with his brother, I was sitting outside with my brother and cousin. I introduced them, and we had a powerful conversation about life, legacy, and purpose. He left me with some simple and moving words that I continue to keep with me today: *Y'all gon be alright, I know y'all are gon' be alright. I'm not worried about that at all.* I remember being floored and grateful for that salute from one of the best musicians who has ever walked.

At that moment, Mr. Isley was serving as a much-needed reflection. That's what infinite possibilities create. They make experiences into full-circle moments. I hadn't seen this man since I was a kid, and to have him affirm me and my existence so strongly was beyond impactful. It was like this random run-in wasn't random at all. I was being shown something in divine timing. Being deeply immersed in my spiritual path, I knew this run-in was not a coincidence. I was being reminded how important it is to maintain a positive attitude and outlook on life even when things are not going as planned. Infinite possibilities create divine timing if we allow it. If we drop our guard and don't get caught up in how we think things should happen but instead accept how things happen, the true beauty and teachings of life will be abundant and bright. In doing so, we open ourselves up to something better and just for us. I left the exchange remembering to walk my path. And trusting that it's okay when folks we thought were meant to be a book in our lives turn out to be only a chapter—because there will always be more space to write and rewrite our personal stories.

The older I get, the more I trust the timing of my life, the more I lean into loss and do-overs with curiosity and awe versus a closed heart and mind. No matter what happens, there's a possibility for a greater outcome and clearer reflections recognized by those who really and truly see us. This is why it's crucial to do your best and not get hung up on how things happen. We cannot control what happens to us in this life, but we can control how we choose to show up and face adversity. Everything won't always pan out how we expect it to and, to me, that has exercised my commitment to being emotionally strong and sound.

Building on my strength has been game changing for me, especially on a spiritual level. It's shown me the importance of realizing what I bring to the table in my career, relationships, and overall life. I also have learned on a deeper level how to see the value of my resilience and understand. Creating a sense of value in our life is sacred and requires being strong-willed enough to commit, even when things feel like they aren't in our favor. This, for me, all comes back to the power of choice and self-belief.

| Energy Check: Infinite Possibilities

What kind of future do you see for yourself?

Do you have the patience that it takes to manifest your wildest dreams?

Are you willing to accept what you need to do in order to improve yourself?

Are you content with your life?

How will you unlock your abundance?

Being realistic about what I bring to the table has catapulted me to a space of spiritual expansion. It's one thing to say you're strong. It's another to take it a step further and put your strengths, whatever they are, into practice.

Reflecting on my career as a whole, it's evident that sometimes my strengths didn't always work out as I envisioned. Taking the good with the bad has afforded me a new sense of open-mindedness. And in my moments of disappointment, I also am equipped with an arsenal of strength. Things shifting doesn't strip me of my power. It offers me a new perspective and a new chance to shift. This process is all a part of the building and re-building. It puts us in a position to trust ourselves more because we're actually building and challenging ourselves to improve. Step-by-step, I shape my greatness. Building on my strengths is critical to me because it's tangible. It's something that I know can support my longevity on all fronts. I'm confident about this because it's allowed me to use my gifts and in better ways, in different ways. It gives a sense of value, especially when I've put the work in. When we do the work, no one can ever take that away.

One of my strengths is my ability to remain positive through life's sometimes hostile and harsh terrain. I take pride in being able to become positive in those moments. This has allowed me to choose who I want to be. It's also really helped me see new perspectives—and it's put me in a position to accept certain things as they are. Acceptance is a choice—one that allows me to build on my strength and my positivity. This mindset has helped me tremendously throughout my career. Especially when I hit a low point with the members of B2K, I became even more grounded in my integrity as a man. I take pride in the fact that the people who I have encountered in life, be it the doorman, a taxi driver, or a colleague, are left with a sliver of happiness from me, one that leaves them holding me in high regard and mutual respect on a human level.

Sometimes as entertainers, we can shy away from day-to-day interactions with people. What I've realized on my path is that we need those connections because it humanizes and normalizes our ability to show up and care for people. Even in my challenges with B2K, I've been able to hold on to wanting to connect with people and not lose sight of my character—even when I was being mistreated and disrespected. I am an evolved version of myself because of it all. No matter what I've been through, my ability to treat people with respect, kindness, and warmth continues to be a great strength.

The exchange I had with Mr. Isley was a great reminder from the Universe that I am aligned with my highest potential and the greater good. It's a superpower to be this way—not everyone can move through the world with this type of demeanor and character. I know people are watching, and I want to encourage them to make the choices to rise even when life gets us down. Through my actions, I want to motivate people to do and be better, just like Mr. Isley did for me. Anytime I've done shows, I'm always saluting everybody because it's so important that people feel acknowledged. Building on that strength has allowed me to see that my energy permeates around the planet. Sometimes people run into me, telling me stories that I don't remember, but they vividly remember, and they're like, I remember you and how kind you were to me. I don't want to lose that, even when the going gets tough. Every step of my path has helped me achieve a sense of gratitude and appreciation toward human life and our existence here on earth.

Thinking about my career as a musician, I've been reflecting on what growth looks like for me and how I will continue to transform. There are so many different layers to my purpose, and that reminder from Ron Isley made it very clear for me. I am committed to my well-being—not just as an artist but as a freethinker, a dancer, a father, and a creative human being. The reinvigorating of purpose requires being aware of what it means to stretch and take on new challenges. A part of my personality gets excited to transition and find a new flow in life. Just like Ron expressed, I am not worried about it, one bit. I am extremely mindful and curious about how I will grow in this next stage of my life.

My Nana has always stressed to me that in this life we should always be learning. This notion keeps me cued into my thought of being open to the infinite possibilities of life. When we stop learning, we stop growing. I don't ever want to stop growing. We are not created to be stagnant. As a student of life, my knowledge will continue to expand and teach me how to be my best self. Adversity cannot and will not stop my growth. I am a believer in the power of choice. And even with the challenges that we all face in this life, I believe that having a positive outlook helps us cope with the daily dynamic of life changes.

Staying stuck in negative thought cycles is a distraction from doing the work required of us to grow and change. I've adopted positivity as a way of life to feel more connected to myself and those around me. Living this way brings on constructive changes in our lives. It doesn't mean shitty things don't happen. It doesn't mean that we will avoid all negativity. But it does serve as a reminder that we are in control of how we choose to see things and let them affect us. In my personal quest, it makes me feel happier and lighter and opens up the pathway to a more successful life experience. Becoming self-aware and dedicated to managing my emotions has yielded an abundant outlook in my life. Living this way has given me the choice to see and experience a new perspective. It is never too late to change and start again. That is the lesson of infinite possibilities—that is the joy. Our overall health is directly linked to our mind and spirit, not just our bodies.

As I unfold into the best version of myself, I choose to remember and believe that I am content, that I give myself room to grow and change as many times as I need to, and in the face of negativity I will remember the grace that positivity offers my life. Being open to infinite possibilities leaves room for us to have faith and explore a more meaningful life experience as a whole. During our time on earth, we should commit to making the best of it, no matter what we are faced with. Do not be one of those people who choose to let their circumstances define them. Rise up has your name on it. We are all capable of being the humans we want to be in this world. It takes effort, time, and commitment, but if you're open to the expansion that possibility has waiting for you, you can do what feels unattainable.

This mindset is what sets us apart. We all have different ideas about what's valuable and what makes us feel best. Making our own choices about what we do is essential because it gives our life meaning. Making choices about what's necessary helps us become more independent and in charge of our lives—one of the most important aspects of life decision-making. Every choice that we make affects our lives in a good or a bad way. The power of choice helps shape us and identify who we are to ourselves and other people. Remember, always, that you get to choose. You get to accept. You get to change and stay open to the infinite possibilities of this life and the time you have on this planet. No matter what you plan in life, you have to leave room for flexibility and change. There will be people and instances that try to stop you from being great. That is not your burden to carry. Your job is to stay focused and committed to your truth. Getting distracted and stuck on what is or isn't happening will keep you from doing the work you were called to do in the world. When distractions emerge, remember who you are and who you intend to be.

There have been moments in my life, especially in my career, when I could have quit and walked away. However, doing so wouldn't have gotten me the outcome I said I wanted. Quitting is easy, and I don't take the easy way out. On your journey, there will be people waiting for you to quit or fail and not fulfill your dreams. It's important that we stay grounded and remember that we weren't born to keep company with misery. If there is anything or anyone in your space fueling doubt, consider leaving them behind. Keep in mind that the universe conspires for your dreams and works to make your desires come true.

I am a true believer in manifestation, and I've seen it work in my life. I remember putting out into the world that I wanted to do a duet with a female artist. Not too long after, Summer Walker invited me to be on her new album *Still Over It*. When I put that into the Universe, I wasn't specific about whom I wanted to work with, and it was beautiful to collaborate with her and to witness manifestation work in my favor. Anyone trying to get in the way of that is not worthy of your time, space, and energy.

To stay focused and have things work in your favor, you must be open to what's ahead. Trying to hold on to things that are beneath or behind you will only create confusion on your path. Stay close to clarity. If you're left feeling confused, it's time to change course. Trusting in and knowing what you want in life can become a reality if you work hard while you're manifesting what you want to bring to fruition. I think it's important to note that failure will happen even when you're working your ass off. That's a part of the game.

This is often a test of do you really want what you say you want—and how hard are you willing to work for it? So like my aligned experience with Ron, me being open to his wisdom, his presence, and his words of affirmation over my life were the reminders I needed to keep moving forward and being curious about what I want out of this experience. It showed me that my hard work has and will continue to pay off. His words of affirmation blessed me, and I will continue to reflect on them as my path changes and evolves into something bigger, better, and deeper.

There are so many things I plan on doing within my life and career. Knowing that other people are watching and rooting me on, and have been for years, is an affirmation to keep going. A major takeaway here for me is that everyone isn't praying for my downfall. Most people are celebrating me and will continue to. Best of all, I am committed to celebrating myself. Keeping this mindset is crucial because life can be turbulent. We will get tested time and time again, sometimes on the same thing multiple times—and even when that is the case, you cannot quit. You may have to reroute and switch up a few times, but throwing in the towel isn't going to elevate you and push you toward the life you want to live. Settling isn't an option when you're destined for greatness. And like Ron Isley so graciously told me when leaving the studio, "Y'all gon be alright, I know y'all are gon' be alright. I'm not worried about that at all."

OKAY, YOU DID THAT.
NOW, WHAT'S NEXT?
YOU CAN'T JUST
SIT AROUND
DOING NOTHING!
PUT YOUR BEST FOOT
FORWARD AND KEEP
PRESSING ON.

Infinite Possibilities Mantra

AUM OM

My best self is my true self.
I unlock.

I take full responsibility for reducing stress in my own life.
I unlock.

I act out love, protection, and kindness.
I unlock.

The best is yet to come.
I unlock.

AUM OM

I am awakening my greatest potential and self-realization.
I unlock.

I remember the gifts that I was born with.
I unlock.

I am accepting responsibility and taking initiative.
I unlock.

I am opening up the door of infinite possibilities.
I unlock.

9

Gratitude Is My Attitude

Gratitude is a balancing tool in my life. It allows me to appreciate what I have, from my ability to do what I love for a living, to the heartbeat in my chest. Through meditation, journaling, and simply being alive, I am able to ground down by giving thanks for another day. Nothing happened in particular that transformed my relationship with gratitude other than choosing to open my eyes and pay closer attention to myself and the world around me. Life is fleeting, and waking up to gratitude was a transformation that felt aligned with who I was growing into. Not every transformation comes with a specific practice or teacher: sometimes we just wake up and start seeing the world through new eyes. You can and will change when you're ready. That is the beauty in the journey. Not taking life for granted is when we can truly start to see gratitude as a daily and easeful practice.

Gratitude is defined as the quality of being thankful, the readiness to show appreciation, and the return to kindness. Looking at being grateful through that lens resonates so deeply with me because it's simple. Gratitude invites us to show up, be human, and focus on the little things in front of us. When we sit back and take a moment to realize those simple things, we can grasp the importance of being grateful and present for the small moments. Sometimes I do a gratitude practice in which I think about life and imagine sitting alone in a garden somewhere and watching a butterfly pass by. Being alive is like this delicate dance that invites us to pay attention and really look at what's in front of us. If we blink, we can miss its beauty. As a father, I often think about how fast my kids are growing up and all the moments in between. Having gratitude for big and little things reminds me that nothing is promised but the transition to return back into the Universe. With that being true for each and every one of us, being grateful for the days I have been given invites me to think beyond this body and my current experience.

Giving thanks for all that we walk through is where true self-awareness lies. When life is showing us things not just about others but also about ourselves, the practice of gratitude allows us to sit back, take a look at our lives, and really be thankful that we are here to learn and experience even when we are faced with challenges. It's also an opportunity to look at where we are and what we've walked through and find peace in the process. For me, it's a reminder to keep moving forward, to keep being open to the miracles that life has to offer. Being grateful is a gift to the soul that allows us to see the beauty in our darkest moments.

| Energy Check: Gratitude Is My Attitude

What are the benefits of having gratitude?

What have others done in your life that you're grateful for?

What makes you laugh or smile lately?

What do you appreciate?

What in nature inspires you and why?

My Nana was first diagnosed with cancer in 2014. She went into remission, and it came back again in 2018. That experience has taught me a lot about being grateful for the time I have with the people I love. Spending time with my Nana loving, sharing, and surrounding myself with her love, spiritual knowledge, family stories, and laughter has highlighted the importance of time and how we invest and spend it. Focusing my energy on creating moments with her and my family that will last a lifetime and create a legacy is valuable. Gratitude enhances relationships and reminds us to pay attention and be in the moment. Watching my Nana smile, tell stories, and share her wisdom is a precious gift that I will be forever blessed by.

I find so much liberation in paying attention to the smallest details and giving thanks for being able to witness them. Having an attitude of gratitude requires a certain level of appreciation. There will be moments when we have to go through things, like a loved one being ill, to see the true gift of being grateful for the time and moments of the now. Something that I constantly keep in mind is that we have the power to find gratitude everywhere—even when we think we're blind to it. When we are truly paying attention to what's happening around us, we can see the goodness overflowing in our lives. We have to be open to seeing and recognizing it, though. This, too, is a practice of mindfulness, being open to the gifts of life. Appreciating the small things in life and the little things that may otherwise be overlooked is how an attitude of gratitude is cultivated. This can amplify positivity in our lives and give us the desire to do and be better. Living in gratitude is inspiring on so many levels. My Nana is grateful for every day she has had and is given on this earth. Watching her stand in her power, even with cancer, is a wake-up call for me to be fully present, in every moment of clarity, love, and beauty.

As I grow and move through this life, I am open to receiving each gift that gratitude offers me, especially the joys of life like watching my Nana dance, make shea butter, cook, and create jewelry. Having a grateful spirit in the highs and lows of life is a reminder that there is always something to see the good in. There is always more to learn and to appreciate. The little things will pass us by if we are not open to seeing them fully. Even our challenges. I've learned so much about being grateful for the not-so-fun experiences of life. As we know, things aren't always great, joyous, and beautiful. And even still, opening our hearts up to see what those adverse moments are trying to teach us is another gratitude gift.

I am most grateful for the knowledge that life has taught me. I've gained so much insight into what success looks like and how we are seen by the world. What matters most to me is how I am seen and felt by the ones closest to me: my Nana, my kids, my mom, my brother, my family. That is what truly matters in my life and in my world. Externally, we get messages about how and who we should be—that can cloud what really matters. It can shift our perspective and blind us from recognizing our true selves. I am grateful that for me, and my life, I've stayed connected to what it means to be present and honest in expression and growth. It's not always easy to do. It takes a commitment to self-awareness to not waiver in the face of adversity and external noise.

HAPPY FOR YOU MEDITATION

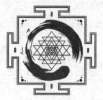

Celebrating others brings happiness and wholeness into my being.

Nine.

When I rejoice with others, I multiply the good times I get to celebrate.

Nine.

I know being a hater is not a good thing.

Nine.

The more I put out, the more I will receive in return.

Nine.

I sincerely congratulate others on their success.

Nine.

I free myself from frustration, worry, and comparisons.

Nine.

I improve my relationships with others by sharing both ups and downs.

Nine.

I look forward to welcoming more joy into my life.

Nine.

The number nine symbolizes divine completeness.

Nine.

In the face of my Nana's illness, I am confronted by how much her life and legacy will continue to shape and teach me long after she's gone. The older I get, and the older she gets, I'm encouraged to sit with her more and learn from her in a new way. Nana and I have a deep history. When I was born, she was the first person to touch me. A practicing doula, she delivered me. And since that day, we have had a bond that is unmatched. My relationship with my Nana is special for a lot of unspoken reasons. How my Nana helped raise us was an example of the trickle-down effect. Growing up, she gave me a vast perspective of life and culture, and I admire her deeply for that. Gratitude flows when I think about how she taught us and continues to teach us, even though my siblings and I are adults. Before I knew myself, my Nana knew me. She knew that I would be a gift in some way—let her tell it.

My Nana tells this story of when my mom got pregnant with me at sixteen. A lot of people around were advocating for an abortion. The first thing Nana said when she heard that was, *We don't kill our own. We show up.* When I heard that story, I was so moved. Because that right there made it clear that she had already spoken for me before I even arrived. Before anyone knew who or what I would be in this world.

I was born on the evening of November 12, a surprise early arrival. My mom was having her baby shower. Nana jokes and says that because I had gotten my gifts, I was ready to get to the party—and since the day I was born, she's been by my side. She is exceptional, not just to me, but to other people. To this day, Nana is revered by kids in the neighborhood my mom grew up in. I'm grateful for the unbreakable bond that I have with my family. It keeps me centered and reminds me of how far I've come. We grew up in a neighborhood that was violent and had a lot of gangs—and my Nana was able to keep us safe and feeling loved through that chaos. There was never a feeling of being unloved. My siblings and I were well protected and shown how to be the best we could be despite our surroundings.

Over the years, I've seen my Nana fight and be a warrior, and she has yet to lose her shit-talking wit, spark, or charisma. Gratitude for the little things is what I see when I look at my Nana and all she's walked through. I've been asking her a lot more questions lately in the midst of her illness to soak up her wisdom and learn from her life experiences. When she talks, I listen. We all do. She mentioned in one of our conversations that life is what we make it. I asked her what she wished someone told her when she was growing up. Her answer was enlightening. She said "to be happy." In her explanation, she shared that happiness is up to us. Everything we do is in our hands.

This wisdom blew my mind and made me even more committed to loving my family and leaning into growth. My Nana got married at seventeen and to hear her say she wished someone told her more about happiness and the power of choice really made me think of how many people do things because they think they have no other choice. Of course, times were different when she was a young woman, but the fact that she intentionally helped raise us to be happy freethinkers is a blessing. Nana is the oldest of eight children, so she had roles and responsibilities that her siblings did not. Listening to her talk, I could tell that she wished some things were different. And maybe she felt like she didn't have a choice when it came to certain experiences. To say I'm grateful for the sacrifices she made for our bloodline would be an understatement. She is the changemaker in our family, the first person to touch me as I entered the world. The one who spoke up for me when I had to be born. There is something special and sacred about that.

My Nana is still just as nurturing and witty as she's always been. She knows I have everything, yet she still asks me if I need anything. If I say no, she'll find something to offer. For as long as I can remember, she's always wanted to give, not just tangible things. Her ability to pay close attention and to offer the gift of her presence and love continues to inspire me. She's special for more reasons than I can count. I know when she leaves this earth, it will be my job to step in, as the oldest grandson, and keep her legacy alive. Nana is one of a kind. I've seen her fight to stay alive, and I've witnessed her perseverance. It's been hard at times, but she always expressed gratitude for life and being able to see another day. One weekend when she was recovering from a chemo treatment, we were sitting outside talking. I remember looking at her small ninety-five-pound frame and thinking how much of a fighter she is. It has been hard for her to eat and keep food down. She was tiny because of cancer but still mighty in her ability to overcome and to be present with us.

Witnessing my Nana growing older has made life and death feel more real to me. I'm reminded that with age comes the deterioration of time. For all of us, it's inevitable that our time on earth will come to an end. Having an attitude of gratitude teaches me to continue growing into the man I was raised to be. I'm the first one in my family to have access to certain things and knowledge. Because of that, my familial generation has it easier than my mom and my grandmother. That is growth. Every stride the folks before us took for the betterment of our lineage blessed me, my siblings, and cousins. Life has taught me that if we don't learn and become better, we will suffocate—it can choke us out and leave us lost. Not learning how to do better and how to live a life that is fulfilling can kill you.

I keep taking notes from the elders in my life. Every chance I get, I ask my Nana questions about her life, lessons, and feelings. It's been interesting to learn that she had to fight for most things in her life. Even now. There have been certain moments where I've wondered if she wanted to quit and give up. If she did, none of us would blame her. Life is hard—but she's never tapped out. She's always stood in her ability to be resilient, even with her fight with cancer.

Everything we face in life is a piece of our realization. All the things we walk through are a part of our experience. The most important takeaway in this phase of my life is sitting down and listening to my elders. To absorb the stories of my Nana while she's still here, to learn from them. That is the trick, paying attention and becoming better while doing it.

Growing up, we all lived together for a while before my mom got her own place. I remember living as a unit so clearly and learning from the women in my life at such a young age. There were moments when I wanted a father figure around, but I'm grateful that things were what and how they were as I reflect on my childhood and my lessons in becoming a man. My life would not be what it is if things were different.

The older I get, the deeper my love and appreciation grows for my Nana. She's such a special lady, and her humor is on point. I could sit and laugh with her all day. I try to memorize her movements when she dances and sings. Her spirit is so vibrant. We all get so much for her. She taught us early on to be seen. She likes to show up and have all eyes on her. You know, she enjoys being seen. And she taught us not to shrink or cower. I have deep gratitude for the examples she set and continues to set for me.

Affirmations for Gratitude

Read these out loud in a seated position.

I am grateful for my breath.

I am grateful for my life.

I am grateful for my beating heart.

I am grateful for my discernment.

I am grateful for my challenges.

I am grateful for releasing what no longer serves me.

I have an attitude of gratitude and I am growing every single day.

I am grateful.

WHAT IT MEANS TO ME: Standing firm in gratitude is a beautiful test of paying attention. I am reminded that every day that I rise is a blessing. I do not take my life for granted. Over the years, I have started paying closer attention to the little things that make me who I am. Being grateful for the highs and lows of life is a reminder that we are alive and blessed. The challenging life moments have taught me so much about myself, and I am grateful for that. The easeful life moments have taught me about appreciating what is in front of me, and I am grateful for that too. Having an attitude of gratitude is a sacred reminder not only to be alive but also to be present.

READER REFLECTION: What are you most grateful for in your life? List your challenges in your journal and pair them with gratitude. List your wins in your journal and pair those with gratitude also. Learn to be thankful for it all; there is a lesson of love and understanding waiting for you on the other side.

As I look back on my life, I am grateful for all the messages that the Universe has given me over the years. I am humbled by listening and paying attention to the signs and wonders of what is around me. I'm grateful that I am able to connect with people and make them feel good through music and dance. I'm humbled by the teachings of my Nana as I've grown into a man who is intentional and purpose driven. Being a medium of music, a son, father, and grandson, I have learned the importance and power of authenticity and freedom. Having an impact on those around me, from my fans to my loved ones, also has a deep and resounding impact on me. I am thankful for the ability to touch lives, listen to others, and bring joy to those I encounter. There is no greater feeling than that.

Everything that has gone wrong and right in my life has been a lesson of perseverance and courage. I give thanks for it all. It all made and shaped me into the man I am today. It's easy to get discouraged and caught up in what we didn't have. But I am committed to seeing and accepting the good of what I did have. Through it all, I've been able to clearly realize my value as an individual and as a member of society. I'm clear about the life I want to live and actualize for myself—that brings me a lot of joy and gratitude. I've been through highs and lows just like everyone else. And as an entertainer, I think folks overlook the humanness of the work I do. I am so much more than an artist and musician. I am so much more than a famous entertainer. I am a son, a dad, a brother, and a man who learned every single day what it means to live in alignment with my highest good, not just for myself but also for those around me. I was raised by women who instilled selflessness in me. They taught me how to show up for others and be accountable for how I move through life.

What continues to give me purpose and commitment to living gratefully is realizing the strength it takes to start over and begin again. I've dropped the ball many times. I've stumbled and got shit wrong a lot. Lessons are born when we hit the ground sometimes. The best thing we can do to course correct is to get back up and try again. Failure comes with life. Success isn't easy to hold on to. There has to be trial, error, and dedication to keep learning and getting better. Something innate inside me stays motivated to wake up every day, start over, and come up with a new plan, idea, or strategy to be the very best version of O that I can be. If my Nana can be the fighter she is, I have no choice but to be a fighter too.

There are no excuses, and for me, being average isn't an option. I come from a bloodline of greatness. Every single day we are blessed with is a new day to start from scratch and create the life you long for. It's a new day to be grateful for all the things you've learned, all the breakthroughs you've had, and all the moments you've been blessed with. My Nana's wisdom allows this to ring true for me. Gratitude, for me, is about shifting perspective and being open to change. Nothing stays the same. Everything changes and takes on a new shape. Being grateful, even for the hard shit, *is* growth. And within the repetitiveness of life, there is a bliss that I am still searching for, one that often brings me back to giving thanks for all that I've grown through and learned from over the years. I continued to be motivated and inspired by people and life and the experiences that I walk through.

Having an attitude of gratitude can change you. It forces you to look closely. It's an invitation to pay very close attention to who you are and who you pray you'll be one day. I'm constantly inspired by the flexibility offered in gratitude. It shows me the importance of stretching my mind to understand new things. We have to be hungry for it. We have to be motivated to open our eyes to see it. We have to be hungry to get fed. That requires determination and dedication to being better than we were yesterday. To be more present than we've been before.

Living this way and thinking how I do has helped me attain inner clarity. Being grateful for every step of my journey has offered me a more present reality—a more confident reality. Not second-guessing myself and allowing doubt, fear, or negativity to pierce my spirit is a daily practice. It brings me back to my attitude of gratitude. Each step in my career and personal life has offered me newfound confidence and courage to manifest and create the life I'm destined to live.

As I've listened to Nana's stories over the years, one of the key things she's expressed is the magic in being decisive and refusing to second-guess yourself when your gut is speaking the truth to you. Intuition is something that offers clarity and deepens my sense of gratitude. Over time, this has put things into perspective. And when things are in view, we become more thoughtful and intentional. When we are willing to accept all that greets us in life, we have a great chance of winning. Everything that we set our mind to, that we think is the right move, won't always be the right move, and even in those moments, there is something to be learned. Over time we discover how to succeed and create abundance by failing. That is why when a situation arrives that can knock us down or throw us for a loop, being decisive and confident can make you feel like you're capable of building the life that you want to live even when adversity strikes.

We won't always get what we want; I've seen and experienced that firsthand. And when that happens—when we lose or stumble—we must be aware and present enough to create room for gratitude and do things differently the next time. Even though specific outcomes weren't what we wanted, there's peace in the knowledge that we can reroute and change course. Moving on is part of my freedom to live in gratitude. As my Nana so often reminds me, it's all up to me. I want to encourage you with those same words. The life you want to live is all up to you. Give thanks for everything you've faced, even if you feel like it's broken you. You're not broken—none of us are.

LEAN INTO THE
WHOLENESS OF YOUR
LIFE AND EXPERIENCES.
BEING PRESENT
WILL TEACH YOU
ABOUT THINGS
THAT ARE GREATER
THAN YOURSELF.

Gratitude Is My Attitude Mantra

At this very moment I am grateful . . .

I am thankful that I have everything that I need.
Thank you.

I am grateful that I have the strength to get through
difficult moments.
Thank you.

I acknowledge and appreciate the divine sanction
placed on my life.
Thank you.

Gratitude brings me in harmony with everything good.
Thank you.

I am grateful for the abundance in my life.
Thank you.

I disrupt anxiety with gratitude.
Thank you.

At this very moment I am grateful . . .
Gratitude is my attitude thank you thank you thank you!

I WILL DO ALL THAT I
CAN TO LIVE IN THE
MOMENT AND NOT
RUSH MY PROCESS.

Letter to My Children

A'mei and Megaa,
When you read this letter years from now, when you're older and able
to understand these words on a deeper level, I hope it leaves you feeling
supported and deeply loved by me. Words cannot express how grateful
I am to be a part of your lives. As your father, I'm honored to share my
knowledge and wisdom with you both. This advice can be applied to all
aspects of your life. Remember them to hold them close.

I want to start by reminding you that you can achieve anything that
you put your mind to. Yes, anything. With hard work, commitment,
and dedication, all that your heart desires can be experienced. Life
is a journey that continues to unfold year after year, experience after
experience. Remember to be present in the moment and have gratitude
for the divine sanction. Everything you encounter will leave you with a
lesson and takeaway if you pay close enough attention. Be true to your-
self always. You are irreplaceable and always enough. Live and thrive
persistently. Trust in yourself and stand firm on your words and stay
forever aligned with the truth—your truth. Purpose, passion, wellness,
family, friends, discernment, and impact of experiences should fill and
overflow your life's cup. Good, bad, or indifferent, respect is the base
foundation to build good things. Realize true lies and separate the
people whose words aren't harmonious with their actions. Hold your
friends and family accountable. Be a truth seeker and never stop learn-
ing. Having respect for yourself and others creates a fair environment.
Be unpredictable. And don't ever forget to pay close attention to the

signals of your gut. Your intuition will lead you if you let it. Channel your emotions. Utilize your strengths. Always keep it real, especially with yourself. My love for you all stretches beyond the cosmos. Our love has no beginning and no end.

All you need to be happy is within you. Many people seek happiness in food, drugs, alcohol, shopping, partying, sex, money, and approval from others because external validation is comforting. What they don't realize is that the tools for happiness aren't outside them. They're within us all. Gratitude, compassion, thoughtfulness, mindfulness, and the ability to create and do something meaningful, even in a nominal way, make life worth living. Happiness lives in the middle of it all. Never stop learning. Have fun, stay active, and be healthy! Never avoid discomfort. Stay ready, so you won't have to get ready. Have a plan. Strategize. You don't need anyone else to make you happy or validate you. You don't need a boyfriend or girlfriend to tell you that you're lovable. You are love, no questions asked. Having loved ones, friends, and family in your life is amazing, and still, you must know and trust who you are. No one else, no matter how much they love you, can do that for you.

Remember to always be yourself. As you mature, make sure you learn to take the necessary time to know yourself and unapologetically be you. Hold yourself and how you treat others in high regard because community is a beautiful thing. Be confident and kind in all that you do. Treat people with honesty, dignity, and respect. There is only one you. You have to be your authentic and entire self. Keep that in mind as you navigate life. Enjoy life as a daily process and practice. Lean into being different and unique. That is what makes you great. Being yourself is a beautiful thing. There may be times where you stray, but you can always find your way back when you stay grounded in your ability to grow and change.

Becoming your father gave me 20/20 vision. Your births shed light on some changes that I needed to make in my life. You both are reflections of that change and growth. You woke up a new person inside of me. Megaa, I remember when you were born, I really got to see what a miracle was for the first time. Seeing you come into the world was surreal and such a revelation of beauty. Having a son made me want to man up and be the very best version of myself. You made me responsible and created room for me to go deep within my experience. No one taught me how to be a dad. No manuscript came with parenthood. In the beginning, I had no idea what I was doing, but having you both as my children made me want to learn and grow in new ways. Learning as you go will be how you figure things out at some points in life. You both brought awareness to my immense focus. Raising you has required me to explore a new version of myself. I did a lot of self-reflecting, and I learned what it meant to do things for myself and others. I hope I've shown you how to be loving, giving, and caring. Being your father is an honor, and fatherhood has helped me immensely become a greater version of myself.

Change is the one constant thing in life. You will suffer trying to hold on to things that you need to grow from. Learn to let go. Find wholeness in releasing what is no longer uplifting your spirit. Continue to meditate and stay close to your inner truth. Keep a flexible mind. Don't get stuck in a rut. Don't shut out what's new and uncomfortable. Try new things and be receptive to new possibilities, especially when things don't go as planned. Be willing to accept the wounds that come with having an open heart. Life is astonishing if you don't shut out the world. Stay curious and flexible. If, at first, you don't succeed, take a beat, then take another crack at it. Trial and error are sacred. Be resilient, have gangster persistence. Stay in touch with Mother Nature. Plant trees. Go on hikes. Ride bikes. Dance forever. Respect the planet. Breathe in the fresh air around you. Remember that you are alive, and that is a blessing to this earth! Help others and take good care of yourselves and each other. Your bond as brother and sister is irreplaceable. Keep things in your life that are in alignment with your purpose. Don't ever doubt how valuable you are. As you grow and evolve, you'll learn that certain things and people won't be able to grow with you. You must be mindful of this part of the journey. Shedding is hard, but we are all made to let go at some point. Don't hold yourself hostage to your mistakes. Apologize when you're wrong. Be kind to yourself when you fail. Everything happens for a reason and in divine time. You don't have to rush anything, because whatever is meant for you will find it's the way. Work hard at the things you love and the things you don't love. Keep your word and finish what you start. Effort counts and is extremely important. Always know, no matter what, I love you with every fiber of my being, and no matter where you go on this life's journey, the essence of my life lives inside of you. You don't have to make me proud, because I already am. Have pride in yourself and stay connected to *your passions, truths, and the infinite possibilities that this life has to offer. Continue to carry it on through the generations to come. Know that I'm with you always. There is not a step you can take where I won't be. Both of you are a gift to my life and the world. Keep being the amazing people you were born to be.*

Love,
Dad, Omari Ishmael Grandberry

I CHOOSE TO SEE THE GOOD IN PEOPLE; I CHOOSE TO SEE EVERYONE'S VALUE, EVEN IF WE DON'T MESH OR AGREE. IT ALL COMES BACK TO CHOICE. I REFUSE TO BE HARDENED BY THE STRUGGLES OF LIFE AND BEING LET DOWN. I CHOOSE TO RISE UP AND REMEMBER WHAT I BRING TO THE TABLE.

10

Relationship with
Rhythm + Spirituality

I am making the connection to life through rhythm.
I dance.

Everything has rhythm. To live is to be musical.
I dance.

Rhythm is the universal language of the soul.
I dance.

I bring balance and order to my life with rhythm and harmony.
I dance.

All emotions are connected to the breath. If you change
the breath and rhythm, you can shift the emotions.
I breathe.

I am a powerful medium when I submit to the rhythm
of my heartbeat.
I listen.

Cadence, flow, patterns, life is but an eternal dance.

My mom was a ballet dancer. While she was pregnant with
me at the precious age of sixteen, she continued to dance and

have music be a major part of her life throughout my childhood. I often say I fell in love with dancing when I was in the
womb. My mom was a dancer and had been for many years
before having me. Even after my birth, she danced. She was
even on *Soul Train*. Dance is embedded in my DNA. That's
when my relationship with rhythm started. I had no choice
but to dance.

Fast-forward to me becoming a father. As I prepared to become a dad, I attended some birthing classes with my doula and
learned the importance and value of playing music for the growing babies inside their mother's womb. That was exciting for
me—being able to play my favorite songs to Megaa and A'mei
from the outside world. That experience was magical and still
leaves me in awe. Knowing that my children could feel and experience the joy of music before coming into the world was exciting for me, as a lover of all things music and movement. Both of
my children, like me, have an innate relationship with rhythm.
And I can only guess that came from introducing them to sound
and the vibration of different types of music before they made
it earthside.

Rhythm has always guided my life. Not just as a performer
but also as a man. Thinking about the different ways it shows up
in my life is striking, from the sound of my heartbeat to the rise
and fall of my lungs while breathing. I am in tune and aligned
with all aspects of how rhythm shows up in my life. And when I
am onstage entertaining and putting on a show, the music takes

over my entire body. This is how I know it is a part of me that I can never escape.

There are moments when I'm dancing where I am no longer just responding to the sounds: I become the expression of the sounds. Over the many years of loving and being a dancer, I have learned to play with rhythm by controlling how I move, breathe, and take on new shapes. When I dance, I get lost in the best way possible. I become the medium of the music and I tap into another essence of my being. Freeness of movement opens up the capacity of my body and my breath that are unlocked with every step. Dancing is a spiritual act for me. It allows me to tap into certain emotions at the right time and explore the journey of becoming a medium of music. Many times when I am dancing, I am present but also not present. I have learned to move and let go of the idea of being in control. Allowing things to just be in flow without force is a practice that I am constantly learning and evolving in. Just like yoga, there are certain positions and moves that open up the capacity of our bodies and breath that have been around for hundreds of years. Dance is similar in the sense that it's another ancient expression for being in tune and in touch with movement, breathing, and creative expression. Dance allows me to unlock things within my body. It reminds me of what is possible and what I am capable of.

The spiritual side of dancing allows me to become quiet and exist in a space that only I can see. I sometimes view the stage as an altar, and I step into a new realm of being. One night on the Millennium Tour it got spiritual for me and everything disappeared. We were in a sold-out arena, fans screaming, music blasting, and I felt like no one was there. It's almost like a pause button was pushed and I left my body. Everything around me stopped. This has happened before, and sometimes it can be a little intimidating and scary. I wear in-ear monitors onstage for extended periods of time. When wearing these, you can't really connect with the natural sounds of the outside world. You can only hear what's going on backstage and soundcheck, which can be an odd experience for nonentertainers.

Walking onstage, I can't hear the crowd but I can see and feel the energy. It's like I'm tethered between two worlds. So when it was time to dance, it felt like I was the only one there. Me, the rhythm of the music, and my heartbeat. I wasn't thinking about where I was stepping or moving. I was just floating and being one with the altar I had created onstage. In those moments, I have to stay in tune with myself. On that night, I was getting carried away. I could feel myself leaving my body more and more. The energy and magic that comes from my spins and everything else in between were taking over. I was married to music at the moment. Bringing myself back to reality is always important because I still have cues, marks, and places to be on the stage. Dancing is very spiritual in that way, where it can take over your entire being. Yes, you want that to happen, but you also must have a healthy relationship with it. You don't want to get so lost where it's like *Damn, I missed my cue because I got carried away.*

| Energy Check: Relationship with Rhythm

How does rhythm affect your daily life?

What is your circadian rhythm?

How important is rhythm?

How important is timing?

What are some benefits you get from dancing?

Exploring the spiritual side of dance continues to teach me how to be a vessel for my craft. Experiencing this on tour night after night is incredible. Especially because every show is different. I'm always *making adjustments* through my freestyle moments to maintain a sense of freeness and originality. From dance to walking, to yoga and stillness—I think there is so much value in everyone moving their body in some way. Dance, for me, is an act of joy and resilience. Life is rhythm. Every breath that we breathe is sustaining us and calls us to move and pay attention. It's essential to realize the rhythm of life and the timing of everything we do. When we're able to create this space of trust and attention in our lives, we begin to move and shift and grow. No matter what we choose to do or how we choose to do it, being fully present in our bodies is necessary for growth, thriving, and emotional expansion.

At all ages, we can find joy and play in the different movements available to us. Whether you're a performer or not, it's beneficial to trust the timing of your life. Creating a routine for your spiritual practices that can also link back to rhythm and its connection to the movement of life. When I'm not dancing or performing, I am finding other ways to recalibrate and reclaim my energy. Traveling all over the world has created space for me to get to know myself on a deeper level.

I found that having a morning routine amplifies my ability to be clear-minded and present. I have a practice of waking up at five in the morning or rising with the sun a day or two a week, which allows me to move slowly and be in a state of presence and mindfulness. Rising early, and before the sun comes up, rejuvenates my energy and reminds me to be in the moments of stillness that I'm offered. Often these early mornings include dancing by myself, for myself. Tapping into this practice helps me not feel all over the place and prepares me to organize my energy and get clear with my thoughts for the day.

Preserving our energy and getting into the rhythm of our lives means we have to sacrifice to get what we want. That may look like waking up at five in the morning, or maybe it means saying no to the things you know do not serve you. Creating a ritual and rhythm in our life is an extension of our growth. All the different rhythms in my life, personal and professional, have helped me manage and preserve my skill set. They've made me a stronger and more aware person and performer, all the way around.

I can't imagine my life without dance, music, and movement. It's my saving grace and a major part of my identity. Being able to find peace and meditation on and off the stage by listening to the beat and feeling the rhythm reminds me to stay attune and present to everything around me. Dance is a teacher that knows no rules and has no obstacles. I am honored to be a student of rhythm and dance. Moving my body liberates me and encourages me to let go and try again. There is nothing permanent about this life, all we have is now. Thanks to my mother's early lessons on movement, I've been experiencing dance since before I could walk and talk. It has been one of her best gifts to me. I've learned how to be my true self, not only as a performer but as a student of this life and craft. There is no greater realization than to see how hard work, dedication, and commitment to your craft can manifest into a life-changing practice.

DANCE IS AN
OUTPOURING OF THE
EXUBERANCE OF ONE'S
LIFE ENERGIES.
WE DO NOT CONSIDER
SOMEBODY DIVINE
OR GODLY UNLESS
THEIR LIFE ENERGIES
ARE EXUBERANT AND
OVERFLOWING.

Sadhguru

| Energy Check: Journal Prompts

Where do you need to create a rhythm in your life?

What practices of movement bring you joy?

How can you clear up your energy to become more present?

Do you trust the timing of your life?

What made you feel like you're the only person in the room?

11

Happiness + Wholeness

I have a unique perspective when it comes to accepting that we are all different and will embark on pathways that will sometimes not align with others. I was woken up to that early in my career. I've been working since I was fourteen. As a young entertainer in the group, we were expected to put everyone's expectations and bottom line first. We were kids working nonstop with a demanding schedule that often didn't us afford us time to play, rest, or eat properly. Through it all, even when life was tough as a B2K member, I never let anything negative that I was going through steal my joy. We were together, nonstop, as a unit so it was my job to move and live accordingly. So when it was time to part ways and embark on journeys that left some folks behind, I found an even deeper connection to my happiness.

Moving on and writing down my thoughts and feelings in my journals was an opportunity for growth and rediscovery. Those lessons soon overflowed into my personal life. Coming to grips with the reality of letting go as a growth practice has allowed me to understand myself deeper and become aligned with acceptance. It taught me that no matter what, happiness is a choice. We can part ways with people and still wish them the best. We can take a different path, not knowing where to turn, and still choose to press forward. There is so much beauty in that. When I think back on my relationship with the other members of B2K, and when I reflect on my relationship with the mother of my children, even the painful memories, I send grace and well wishes to them. I'm a big believer in people being happy even if that means I am no longer a part of their stories and they are no longer a part of mine.

I am a believer in my power to choose and my commitment to joy. Outgrowing is necessary for us to expand into what truly is meant for us and our lives—both physically and emotionally. So often, we are taught to think that just because we part ways, or our relationship with a person ends, that it automatically means there is beef. While that is the case in some instances, it doesn't have to be long-standing. Parting ways does not have to define us, and we can wish people well when we disconnect from them.

Putting pride and ego aside showed me that our life experiences don't always have to be deep and complicated. Sometimes shit just is what it is. And moving on can be the biggest blessing in disguise. Don't get me wrong, I went through real betrayal and hurtful shit with the mother of my children and my former bandmate. But I also deeply understand and realize that my emotional well-being required that I let them and all ill feelings associated with them go. I choose peace of mind, which in turn gave me happiness and a feeling of completion.

Allowing people to leech off my high vibrational energy is never an option, nor was it conducive to my growth as a man. I've committed myself to be a man of forgiveness, and it's important to me that I not only lead by example but that I live by example too. I release all grudges to gain emotional freedom. While there have been quite a few people over the years that have done me wrong. I sincerely wish them nothing but happiness. I hope they sleep well and feel nourished by life. I hope they feel fulfilled and satisfied on their path—and if they don't, I hope they get there. We all deserve that.

I know people look at me like I'm either crazy, faking it, or the most Zen dude of all time. I am none of the above. I am, however, open to the teachings of life. If I wasn't open to this, I would be stuck in a cycle of hurt and unhappiness, and that is never the goal. I am choosing not to be or stay stuck. That serves no one. Our personal happiness and wholeness is up to us and us alone. No one can make us happy on a holistic level. No one makes us whole either. We are the gurus of our own lives and existence. Trusting in this allowed a new type of growth to happen in my life. The blessings in moving on are liberating.

Affirmations for Peace

Read these out loud in a seated position.

I am worthy of a clear and peaceful mind.

I am open to healing.

I am trusting the timing of my life.

I am committed to handling my business and staying on track.

WHAT IT MEANS TO ME: I believe that peace is an energetic currency. We have to be mindful of how we spend our time and how we invest it. Our peace can either be drained or be replenished. It's important that we make time and space for things that fuel us and bring ease to our life. Even in moments of adversity, I believe that we can find and secure our peace. We are in charge of where our energy goes and flows. Stay open to the possibilities and the timing of life, our peace will flow freely if we allow it.

READER REFLECTION: What brings you peace of mind? Create a list that reminds you of the things that bring you calming energy. Commit to practicing them daily and keeping your vibration elevated in a peaceful state.

Everyone doesn't have the capacity to think differently. We cannot force anyone to see things how we see them. We can only lead by example so that people can bear witness to us and, in turn, learn something. Responding to adversity with attunement versus aggression: that takeaway has taught me so much about individuality and the power of choice that I so deeply believe in. My happiness and wholeness don't depend on how others treat me. I feel that not holding grudges, and instead focusing on my happiness and wholeness, has allowed me to keep my focus sharp. In my development as a man, I've cherished and held fast to my joy because if I didn't, someone or something will try to take it from me—and I've worked too hard to allow that to happen. Releasing grudges is imperative because if not, it becomes a part of our life force, like an extra piece of invisible luggage that we carry around. There are levels to it all, this life.

Over time, the Universe has shown me the importance of continuing on the path of liberating myself, even when that includes leaving people and their mess behind. Letting go of the projected pain of others has given me the opportunity to imprint, impress, and affect those watching and observing. That's why I carry myself the way I do. It's not a temporary act: it's a lifestyle. I feel that's why so many people were so enamored by how I interacted with the unnecessary drama on the Millennium Tour. A lot of folks said, "Nah, fuck them." But for me and my energy, that wasn't going to enrich or raise my vibration.

Our energy and message is transformed into gifts and insight when we commit to healthy happiness versus toxic happiness. Toxic happiness would be saying "Yea, you're right fuck them" and enjoying watching the fall and demise of those who hurt us. That is not aligned with who I am or how I operate. I do not find joy in other people's pain and suffering, although the occasional I told you so pops into mind. I find joy in witnessing their healing and emotional growth. What I don't think a lot of people quite get is the liberation that comes with being genuinely happy for people. I am emotionally free, peaceful, and happy. And I want people, even those who are no longer walking through life with me, to be the same. This is an obstacle of life, and it doesn't have to be a negative one. For me, these obstacles mean that we must evolve into a higher way of being and living.

Facing adversity and hurdles and moving through them to move on is powerful. On a spiritual level, it is a sacred thing. As I continue to evolve, my path to happiness is the way to wholeness. As I become more dedicated to being a man of peace, wisdom, and emotional freedom, liberation finds me. Happiness is a choice. I will continue to connect with my power, honesty, and responsibility by walking through life courageously. Being honorable and honest in the work I do as a performer and black man in the world is something worth nurturing and protecting fiercely. This life is short and is worth living to the fullest. I don't take one single day that I am gifted for granted. And because of that, I can exist as my fullest and true self even when I face challenges, hurt, or hatred.

It's not my job to get people to understand why I am the way I am. Or why I choose happiness and wholeness over drama and brokenness. There is enough of that in the world. Something to remember: everyone isn't going to understand their role in your life. Everyone isn't going to part ways with grace and love. There will be people you encounter who will not rest until they see you broken down. My advice, now and always, is to stay whole and connected. Stay true to yourself and your choices. Don't give anyone the power to break you down—ever. Realize who you are as an individual. Stay close to your truth and character. Doing so paves the way for others. When we think about it, living this way is greater than you and me combined. It is a collective and universal act. We are all integral parts of each other's stories. Our relationships with others are essential in life, even if they don't grow as planned. That's cool to me. It can show us something greater than ourselves, and that builds authenticity and character for the long haul. Creating your happiness and wholeness isn't temporary; it's a forever work in progress. You must stay on your path.

WE ALL RETURN TO THE SOURCE. IN THE END, I WILL COME HOME TO MYSELF.

Looking back must also be an option; that's how we learn. That is how we become better in this life. The learning from our lessons, past relationships, mistakes, and more make room for deeper clarity. They say don't look back. I say don't overlook it. I've grown so much as a man over the years. Getting curious about what happiness means to me, about what I want and need in my relationships, meant looking back at the shortcomings, the low points, and the relationships that didn't last.

I've found balance and harmony in reflection. Throughout all of my transitions, I've heard from people that they'll never look back and I shouldn't either. I get it. It can be uncomfortable to look at our pasts and reflect on how unhappy we have been or how broken we may have felt. But we must. If we are called to look behind us, we should because that is the Universe, God, or whichever higher power you believe in tapping you on the shoulder for a reminder. Paying attention to those signs is necessary to become the people we want to be. There's always another aspect of doing that. There's always another way to look at what's in front of us or behind us.

Our pasts are filled with gems that we haven't yet unearthed. Ignoring them doesn't mean they vanish. What I've realized is that choosing not to look back is a passive way of saying I am okay with the past, even when we may not be. As I mature, I feel so much resilience in saying to myself that if I need to go back and dig up or address something, I am more than okay with it. I would rather that than to stay unsettled, unhappy, and unclear. Wholeness requires looking at the pieces in front of us. There's a power in and acceptance of it all.

| Energy Check: Happiness + Wholeness

How can forgiveness allow you to wish someone well who has once caused you pain genuinely?

Are happy people more successful?

What is the importance of being stress-free?

Are happy people healthier in life?

Do you have the courage to kill negativity with happiness?

Many times when I was walking through a very public situation with the mother of my children, people tried to dictate how I should be because they didn't understand that I was choosing to take the higher road. I get that not everyone is me, but learn from that fact. Not everyone is you; take the higher roads of your life. Accept the changing of paths. Be open to the reroutes ahead, because there will be plenty. Don't be swayed by your struggles. You will have intense moments of fear, failure, and uncertainty along your journey. Instead of turning away from those things, turn toward them. Let the hard moments in your life guide you to your highest self.

Happiness is waiting for you, but you have to choose it. You have to want it badly enough to chase it when you feel like you can't. Be the person who you wished you had been growing up. Be the change and live in alignment with your highest good. You get to decide how you want to live. There is power in realizing the importance of moving through the world in this way. It's easier said than done. People will try us, push our buttons, hurt us intentionally, and try to steal the very joy we worked so hard for. Trying to prove them wrong or investing your energy in trying to get them to stop isn't the best use of your sacred time.

You are whole even when folks would rather see you in pieces. Everything you walk through is preparing you for abundance. I can see that more clearly now. There were moments when I was touring with B2K, thinking what am I still doing here. But I knew that there was something greater in store for me and for them. I knew that going backward was my way of moving forward. There are a lot of things that outsiders will never understand about your life or choices, especially as it pertains to your true self and happiness.

Try not to get blinded or bogged down by being misunderstood. That's a part of life. It's a test to show the Universe and yourself that you are who you say you are. When shit gets hard or feels heavy, commit to trusting that you are right where you need to be, and so are the other people who are a part of your story.

Sometimes we have to be down and out to figure out where exactly it is we need to be. This teaches us how to stand up for ourselves and protect what is divinely ours. Recognize who you are no matter what. Growing up in the entertainment industry, I was taught, by watching, early on that if you don't know who you are no one will know who you are. And folks will try to mold you into the version of you they think you should be. That's no way to live. So as you embark on this journey of happiness, remember the beauty in knowing your damn self. Owning your truth and never allowing anyone to steal your happiness. You are a work in progress and a work of art, even with your flaws. Being whole is not about anyone else but you.

We have to remember that we are the common denominator in our lives. It's easy to lose sight of that when things feel heavy. But it's important to remember that weight builds strength, and it's a reminder that we can and will persevere. Invest time in loving yourself and being your own inspiration. The hardships we face are setting us up for beautiful lessons. There may be moments when it's challenging to see it that way. No one said this journey would be easy. Keep going, keep growing, and keep connecting to the inner source that is you.

JUST BECAUSE I GOT MY HEART BROKEN DOESN'T MEAN I DON'T DESERVE A NEW EXPERIENCE. STEPPING BACK TO LOOK AT OUR FULL EXPERIENCE ALLOWS US A CHOICE TO CHANGE AND MOVE FORWARD.

Affirmations for Love

Read these out loud in a seated position.

I am worthy of love.

I can create the love I want for myself in my life.

My heartbreak has taught me the importance of self-love.

I will devote my time and energy to loving spaces.

WHAT IT MEANS TO ME: The hurt of past relationships doesn't get to speak for the love we deserve. I believe that we all deserve full loving energy that is healthy, supportive, and warm. Other people not knowing how to love us isn't permission to give up on love all together. It's easy to let the defeat of pain, heartache, and disappointment speak louder than self-love. This affirmation of love reminds me to love myself and learn how to love others better. I will not let any pain from my past hold me back.

READER REFLECTION: Think of a hurtful time in your life, and instead of harboring ill feelings about it, think of a way to greet with love. What has hurt, pain, or heartbreak taught you? How can you take those lessons and turn them into self-love? Take notes on this reflection in your journal.

Affirmations for Self-Trust

Read these out loud in a seated position.

I can trust myself.

At my core, I know what I want in life.

Trusting my gut is in my favor.

I will learn how to be more trusting of myself
over time.

WHAT IT MEANS TO ME: Self-trust is the gateway to inner knowing. I believe that we all know and have our answers. The world teaches us that everyone else knows what's best for us. I do not agree. My intuition guides and leads me. Every day is a practice of learning how to better myself and trust my higher knowledge. This is something that takes time, practice, and dedication. Get to know yourself!

READER REFLECTION: Who taught you what you know? What is true for you and your life? In your journal, write a letter to yourself about trusting your highest self even when it feels scary. Give yourself permission to unwind on the pages to be honest with yourself about who you are and what you want. No one has your answers but you, remember that.

Affirmations for Becoming Your Best

Read these out loud in a seated position.

I am growing into my best self.

I am healing into my best self.

I am working on being my best self.

I show love to myself as I become my best.

WHAT IT MEANS TO ME: I believe that working to become our best self will be an ever-evolving process. It will not happen overnight. These words remind me that I am all that I am. That each step in my life is me marching toward my best self. I am a student of becoming my best. I am committed, so whenever I forget, I can look at these affirmations and remind myself that I am on the right path and headed in the right direction. No matter what, I will stay dedicated and determined to be the best version of myself and the best man I can be. As time goes on, life shows us where we need to improve. Becoming is an opportunity to evolve and expand spiritually and emotionally. Staying on this journey has kept me emotionally sound and connected to my truth.

READER REFLECTION: In your journals, think about who you want to become in this life and write it all down. Don't worry about it sounding too big or too small, just reflect. What is bringing you closer to becoming your best and highest self? Think about what's holding you back. Your life is yours to adjust: stand in your power and don't hold back.

Five Acts of Peace (self-expression)

Below are some practices that I use to stay grounded in peace. A peaceful mindset allows me to be productive and in tune with what matters. I'm sharing a few acts of peace with you below. These methods support me in being fully present in my life. They remind me to pay attention and be open to the life and experiences around me. The little things and shifts in life can really make a difference in how we see the world and how the world sees us. I'd like you to think about your five acts of peace. What brings you calm, joy, and recentering energy? When we stop and think about these things, we start to shift and change our behavior and find our flow in life. Grab your journal and jot down the things that offer you peace, community, and self-expression. Take a look at the little things and work your way out. We are all worthy of peace and inner clarity. I hope this exercise brings you closer to a daily practice of ease.

SAYING THANK YOU WITH A SMILE: While this may seem like a small thing, it's actually a major key to living a peaceful life and spreading peace to others. You never know what people may be going through. Sharing a smile can change someone's entire day and mood. Peace isn't just about the self; it's also about pouring into our community too. We have the power to lift people's spirits with our joy, body language, and kindness.

HELPING SOMEONE LESS FORTUNATE: This has helped create a clearer perspective for me in my life. A lot of things are happening that we have no control over or have any idea about. Being able to show up and help someone, with no strings attached, creates room for community care and brotherhood. The special thing about helping others is that our actions act as a mirror and so does the ability to receive. It's a two-way street. I believe that whatever we may have in abundance, it is our duty to share. Not just monetarily but energetically as well.

ENCOURAGING PEOPLE WE LOVE: Encouragement is sacred and special. It's tied to the ability to realize and recognize those around us. Sharing words of encouragement and affirmation offers inner peace and external peace. It also builds bonds with those we love and serves as a reminder to be there for one another. Doing so offers a sense of ease and peace of mind.

DOING AN UNPLEASANT CHORE WITHOUT COMPLAINING: We all know that no one wants to do what they don't want to do. However, putting off things doesn't make our responsibilities vanish.

Procrastination robs us from our peace. Doing the thing we don't want to do not only teaches us lessons of responsibility but also restores peace in our lives. To be whole and present, we have to learn to move with the punches of life and handle our business.

MOVING YOUR BODY: Surrendering to the movement and rhythm, this serves as a recalibration of peace. When I'm dancing, I create motion that energizes me and brings me into a state of deep peace. Moving our bodies, be it dancing, walking, or stretching, helps us open up our minds to ease and calm.

Don't Second-Guess Yourself (reflection)

Being able to be decisive allows you to stand steadfast in your choices and allows you to take a step back and really be sure about what it is that you want to do. And being decisive puts you in that alignment with whatever decisions you make and not second-guessing yourself. You're in a better position because you've thought out your plan. Being decisive and not second-guessing yourself really helps you build self-trust and self-confidence. Second-guessing yourself makes more room for doubt, worry, and a lot of things that can take you away from the focus of trusting yourself and ease. Being decisive is important to me because when I have to make important decisions, I can do so with confidence in my choices. I was able to take my time and really pay attention to the choices I was making. This helped me see a clear path and aligned outcome.

Most of the time, I've had positive experiences with the practice of being sure of myself and not doubting my mind, heart, and gut. Being self-assured is valuable and important to me so that I can explore the positive outcomes with clarity. In a way, this goes hand and hand with manifestation. We cannot doubt our power and still expect the things in life that we want to come to fruition. We had to stand tall and secure.

As I've matured, I've gotten better at using my self-confidence in every choice that I make. I always ask myself the hard questions before pressing forward. I always weigh my options, and as a man, I think this is essential to being a true leader. I often ask myself, *If you choose this, will it affect something else in your life?* Everything comes full circle, so practicing mindfulness is essential to how we move and show up in the world. If I decide that I want to do something, weighing all my options helps me recognize and get in contact with the part of myself that is most attuned and aligned. I'm constantly reflecting on the needs of my heart and mind. I use being decisive and not second-guessing myself as a marker and a moment of clarity and surety because every ounce of me needs to be present when making a choice. Getting out of pocket isn't an option.

Moving through the world in this way helps me accomplish a more present reality. It allows me to not allow negative thoughts or doubt to pierce my aura and throw me off track. Not allowing myself to be sucked in by fear or negativity protects my energy and keeps my mind sharp. When thinking about how valuable it is to not be swayed by indecisiveness, I've also started to think more about the power and resilience it takes to stand confidently behind the choices we make. Building on that strength is so important because we have to realize how we are showing up and what we are bringing to the table. Being able to understand what you bring to the table, no matter the setting, creates a sense of value for yourself.

Some people have a delusion of what they bring to the table, and that's why it's so essential to build on your strengths and know who you are. You can have talents and abilities, but you've got to be able to take it further. Action has to match your words. Sometimes our strengths aren't even, and they won't always work out as we envision. There is a major key and lesson to take away from that. Being sure of ourselves and standing tall in our resilience makes room for self-trust in our lives. It's an invitation to grow in new and profound ways. When we pay attention to our power, to our flaws, and to our strengths, we are able to be more clear about who we are in the world, in the face of adversity or self-doubt. We can become a master of ourselves in this practice.

Building on my strengths is important to me because it is tangible. It's something that I'm confident about, and building on it will allow me to use my gifts and in better ways—in different ways. It gives me a sense of value, especially when I think back to all the work I've put in. No one can ever take that away from me, and deciding to listen and trust my intuition life gave me a gift of openness, even through adversity.

One of my strengths is my ability to remain positive through negative and harsh terrain and realities. That's allowed me to choose who I want to be. It's also helped me see new perspectives and put me in a position to accept certain things as they are. Acceptance is a choice and one that allows me to build on my strength and my positivity. Second-guessing myself doesn't get me to where I want to go. It won't shape my life for the better. I like to use moments of uncertainty as a time to train myself to reshape my narrative and become better.

Affirmations for a Clear Mind

Read these out loud in a seated position.

My mind is open.

My mind is free.

Mindful of what I let go and release from my conscious thoughts.

My mind is open.

My mind is free.

I will not allow distractions to take me away from my peace.

I am clear headed and driven to be my best self.

WHAT IT MEANS TO ME: Clarity is one of the key factors that can make the difference between failure and success. The more knowledge and wisdom I seek, the more mental clarity I gain.

READER REFLECTION: Asking yourself the right questions can stimulate thought, reflectivity, and further understanding. Write down three questions that you can ask yourself for clarity

EVERYTHING COMES FULL CIRCLE. REMEMBER, BE UNBOTHERED AND CHOOSE THE POWER OF JOY!

ACKNOWLEDGMENTS

The stories and perspectives shared in this book are my contribution and spiritual duty toward the elevation and rise of a conscious planet. Throughout all of my experiences, good or bad, gratitude is my attitude. Sharing our stories empowers our ability to have an appreciation for truth and self-recognition. We all play an individual and collective role in this human experience. Choose your dynamics. Be balanced. Know your role and play it well.

This book is dedicated to my family. Nana, thank you for loving the way you did. I miss you and I will see you on the other side. I would also like to acknowledge my spiritual teachers who in so many ways have enriched my life and shared tools that have expanded my willingness to grow, do the work, and share with the world. Michael Beckwith, thank you for embracing me and supporting my spiritual journey. Agape love. Sadhguru, thank you for inner engineering, Isha, encouraging my spiritual journey and coming all the way to Inglewood, California, from

India! Sri Master Gano Grills, much love for edifying and expanding my spiritual growth. You've empowered me, Galightigus. Alex Elle, thank you for helping me give my words life. To the CAA team, we did it! A special thanks to Anna Paustenbach and the entire HarperOne team for believing in me and this important body of work. Love and gratitude to everyone who contributed to this amazing book. It has been a pleasure!

—*O.*

ABOUT THE AUTHOR

Omarion is a Grammy Award–nominated singer, songwriter, performer, and actor who rose to popularity in the 2000s. As the lead singer of the iconic R&B boy band B2K, he has achieved numerous multiplatinum, chart-topping hits both as the lead singer of B2K and as a solo artist. Omarion has two children and lives in Los Angeles. Visit him at OmarionWorldwide.com.